The 6 Ds of Fecal Microbiota Transplantation

A Primer From Decision to Discharge and Beyond

T0131094

The 6 Ds of Fecal Microbiota Transplantation

A Primer From Decision to Discharge and Beyond

Editors

Jessica R. Allegretti, MD, MPH
Director
Fecal Microbiota Transplant Program
Brigham and Women's Hospital
Harvard Medical School
Boston, Massachusetts

Zain Kassam, MD, MPH
Chief Medical Officer
Finch Therapeutics
Somerville, Massachusetts

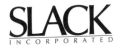

SLACK
INCORPORATED

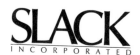

Senior Vice President: Stephanie Arasim Portnoy
Vice President, Editorial: Jennifer Kilpatrick
Vice President, Marketing: Mary Sasso
Acquisitions Editor: Julia Dolinger
Director of Editorial Operations: Jennifer Cahill
Creative Director: Thomas Cavallaro
Cover Artist: Lori Shields
Project Editor: Emily Densten

SLACK Incorporated
6900 Grove Road
Thorofare, NJ 08086 USA
856-848-1000   Fax: 856-848-6091
www.slackbooks.com
© 2021 by SLACK Incorporated

The procedures and practices described in this publication should be implemented in a manner consistent with the professional standards set for the circumstances that apply in each specific situation. Every effort has been made to confirm the accuracy of the information presented and to correctly relate generally accepted practices. The authors, editors, and publisher cannot accept responsibility for errors or exclusions or for the outcome of the material presented herein. There is no expressed or implied warranty of this book or information imparted by it. Care has been taken to ensure that drug selection and dosages are in accordance with currently accepted/recommended practice. Off-label uses of drugs may be discussed. Due to continuing research, changes in government policy and regulations, and various effects of drug reactions and interactions, it is recommended that the reader carefully review all materials and literature provided for each drug, especially those that are new or not frequently used. Some drugs or devices in this publication have clearance for use in a restricted research setting by the Food and Drug Administration or FDA. Each professional should determine the FDA status of any drug or device prior to use in their practice.

Any review or mention of specific companies or products is not intended as an endorsement by the author or publisher.

SLACK Incorporated uses a review process to evaluate submitted material. Prior to publication, educators or clinicians provide important feedback on the content that we publish. We welcome feedback on this work.

Library of Congress Cataloging-in-Publication Data

Names: Allegretti, Jessica R., editor. | Kassam, Zain, editor.

Title: The 6 Ds of fecal microbiota transplantation : a primer from decision to discharge and beyond / editors, Jessica R. Allegretti, Zain Kassam.

Other titles: Six Ds of fecal microbiota transplantation

Description: Thorofare, NJ : SLACK Incorporated, [2021] | Includes bibliographical references and index.

Identifiers: LCCN 2020043899 (print) | LCCN 2020043900 (ebook) | ISBN 9781630917500 (paperback) | ISBN 9781630917517 (epub) | ISBN 9781630917524 (web)

Subjects: MESH: Fecal Microbiota Transplantation | Feces--microbiology | Clostridium Infections--therapy

Classification: LCC QP159 (print) | LCC QP159 (ebook) | NLM WB 365 | DDC 612.3/6--dc23

LC record available at https://lccn.loc.gov/2020043899

LC ebook record available at https://lccn.loc.gov/2020043900

Printed in the United States of America.

Last digit is print number: 10 9 8 7 6 5 4 3 2 1

Dedication

For my husband Andrew, who bought the first blender and whose editing skills are second to none.

—JRA

In memory of my mother, Shaida Kassam, the inspiration for an adventure through uncharted waters.

—ZK

Contents

Acknowledgments

We would like to thank the following:

- All of the contributing authors for pioneering the exciting field of microbiome therapeutics
- All our patients who have trusted us and for participating in clinical trials
- The team at SLACK Incorporated for their support in sharing our vision

Jessica would also like to thank the following:

- First and foremost Zain: thank you for always understanding me and for being the only person who would tolerate writing a book with me. I wouldn't have done it with anyone else.
- My parents, thank you for pushing me to never settle.
- Every current member and alumni of the Allegretti Lab: Maggie, Maddie, J-Mo, Ami, Jenna, Emma, Hannah, Jen, Jonathan, and Jordan. Thank you for making the dream a reality and for scooping all the poop.
- And because once is not enough, to my husband, Andrew, thank you for never letting my think my dreams were too big and for being the best hype man in the biz. I love you.

Zain would also like to thank the following who have helped him through this journey through uncharted waters:

- The builders: Mark Smith, James Burgess, Andrew Noh, Carolyn Edelstein, and all my teammates. Thank you for the courage to dream boldly together.
- The lighthouses: Drs. Paul Moayyedi, Richard Hunt, Eric Alm, and Parveen Wasi. When I lost my way, thanks for shining light on the path forward.
- The engines: Mike Wan, Ian Mak, Thileep Kandasamy, Kanchana Amaratunga. Thanks for helping me discover that it's passion that drives the ship.

- My crew:
  - Lucy, thanks for not letting me get too high or too low as winds change.
  - Faazil, thanks for being a compass, helping me focus on what matters.
  - Dad, thanks for teaching me about the power of purpose.
- To my co-captain: Jessica, thank you for always understanding me and for being the only person who would tolerate writing a book with me. I wouldn't have done it with anyone else.

About the Editors

Jessica R. Allegretti, MD, MPH serves as the Associate Director of the Crohn's and Colitis Center at Brigham and Women's Hospital, Boston, Massachusetts, where she built and leads the Clinical Trials Program. She also founded the hospital's Fecal Microbiota Transplantation Program and continues to serve as the program's Director.

Dr. Allegretti is a gastroenterologist and physician-scientist dedicated to discovering and developing innovative microbiome therapeutics and novel treatments for inflammatory bowel disease. She was awarded the IBD Rising Star Award by the New Chapter of the Crohn's and Colitis Foundation her first year on staff. She serves on the Scientific Advisory Board for OpenBiome, the largest not-for-profit stool bank, and is the Clinical Development Lead for the Massachusetts-Host Microbiome Center. She has authored more than 100 abstracts and peer-reviewed publications in leading journals such as the *New England Journal of Medicine*, *The Lancet*, and *Gastroenterology*, and was recently appointed as an Associate Editor for the *Inflammatory Bowel Diseases Journal*.

Dr. Allegretti has led multiple prospective microbiome therapeutic studies, including the first trials in primary sclerosing cholangitis and obesity. She has received funding from the National Institutes of Health, the American College of Gastroenterology, and the Crohn's and Colitis Foundation. Dr. Allegretti has been featured on HBO, BBC, Netflix, the *New York Times* and numerous other media outlets.

Dr. Allegretti was awarded her MD from the University of Miami. She completed her Internal Medicine training at Massachusetts General Hospital and her GI training at Brigham and Women's Hospital. She went on to receive an MPH degree from the Harvard School of Public Health in Clinical Effectiveness, with a focus on clinical trials.

In 2020, Dr. Allegretti received the Sherman Emerging Leader Prize for Excellence in Crohn's and Colitis and Healio *Gastroenterology*'s Clinical Innovation Award for her work on microbial therapeutics.

Zain Kassam, MD, MPH is Co-Founder and Chief Medical Officer at Finch Therapeutics, a clinical-stage company focused on developing novel microbiome therapeutics. Previously, he was a founding team member and Chief Medical Officer at OpenBiome, the world's first public stool bank for fecal microbiota transplantation, where he helped pioneer the universal donor model and expand safe access to patients suffering from *Clostridioides difficile* infection.

Dr. Kassam is a gastroenterologist, physician-scientist, and biotechnology entrepreneur dedicated to discovering and developing innovative microbiome therapeutics. He was named to the Top 40 Under 40 Healthcare Innovator List by MedTech and received the 2020 Public Health Innovator Award from the Harvard T.H. Chan School of Public Health. Dr. Kassam has served as a Scientific Advisory Board member for the American Gastroenterological Association Center for Gut Microbiome Research and Education, and as a Clinical Research Affiliate at the MIT Center for Microbiome Informatics and Therapeutics. He has authored more than 180 peer-reviewed publications, abstracts, and book chapters, including in leading journals such as the *New England Journal of Medicine*, *Gastroenterology*, and *Gut*.

Dr. Kassam has been involved in more than 25 prospective microbiome therapeutic studies, including the first randomized trials in ulcerative colitis and hepatic encephalopathy. He has held funding from the Centers for Disease Control and Prevention, the Crohn's and Colitis Foundation of America, and numerous private foundations. Dr. Kassam has been featured on PBS, CNN, BBC, *The New Yorker*, *The Washington Post*, and numerous other media outlets.

Dr. Kassam received his MPH degree from Harvard University in Quantitative Methods and completed his post-doctoral training in microbiome engineering at MIT. He was awarded his MD from Western University in London, Canada, where he received the Young Alumni Award for his contributions to the microbiome field. Dr. Kassam completed his Internal Medicine and Gastroenterology training at McMaster University, Hamilton, Ontario, Canada, where he was both the Chief Medical and Chief Gastroenterology Resident.

Contributing Authors

Chathur Acharya, MD
Fellow
Division of Gastroenterology, Hepatology and Nutrition
Virginia Commonwealth University
McGuire VA Medical Center
Richmond, Virginia

Olga C. Aroniadis, MD, MSc
Associate Professor of Clinical Medicine
Division of Gastroenterology and Hepatology
Renaissance School of Medicine at Stony Brook University
Stony Brook, New York

Jasmohan S. Bajaj, MD, MS
Professor of Medicine
Division of Gastroenterology, Hepatology and Nutrition
Virginia Commonwealth University
Central Virginia Veterans Healthcare System
Richmond, Virginia

Thomas J. Borody, MD, PhD, DSc
Professor
Centre for Digestive Diseases
Five Dock, New South Wales, Australia

Lawrence J. Brandt, MD, MACG, AGAF, FASGE
Professor of Medicine and Surgery
Albert Einstein College of Medicine
Emeritus Chief of Gastroenterology
Montefiore Medical Center
Bronx, New York

Shrish Budree, MBChB, DCH, FCPaeds, Cert. Paeds Gastro.
Medical Director
Finch Therapeutics
Somerville, Massachusetts
Guest Lecturer
Faculty of Medicine
University of Cape Town
Cape Town, South Africa

Jennifer D. Claytor, MD, MS
Resident Physician
Department of Internal Medicine
University of California San Francisco
San Francisco, California

Suzanne Devkota, PhD
Assistant Professor
Karsh Division of Gastroenterology and Hepatology
Cedars-Sinai Medical Center
Los Angeles, California

Najwa El-Nachef, MD
Associate Professor
Clinical Medicine
Co-Director
Microbial Restoration Therapy Program
Gastroenterology Fellowship Director
University of California San Francisco
San Francisco, California

Paul Feuerstadt, MD, FACG, AGAF
Assistant Clinical Professor
Yale University School of Medicine
New Haven, Connecticut
PACT Gastroenterology Center
Hamden, Connecticut

Monika Fischer, MD, MSc
Associate Professor of Medicine
IU Health University Hospital
Indianapolis, Indiana

Rohma Ghani, MBBS, MRCP
Infectious Diseases and Microbiology Specialist Registrar
Division of Digestive Diseases
Department of Metabolism, Digestion and Reproduction
Faculty of Medicine
Imperial College London
London, United Kingdom

Ari M. Grinspan, MD
Associate Professor of Medicine
Director of GI Microbial Therapeutics
Department of Medicine
Division of Gastroenterology
Icahn School of Medicine
Mount Sinai Hospital
New York, New York

Lauren Tal Grinspan, MD, PhD
Fellow
Department of Medicine
Division of Gastroenterology
Icahn School of Medicine
Mount Sinai Hospital
New York, New York

Anoja W. Gunaratne, BAMS (Hon), MSc, PhD
Clinical Research Officer
Centre for Digestive Diseases
Five Dock, New South Wales, Australia

Colleen R. Kelly, MD
Associate Professor of Medicine
Department of Medicine
Warren Alpert Medical School of Brown University
Providence, Rhode Island

Alexander Khoruts, MD
Director
Department of Medicine
Division of Gastroenterology, Hepatology, and Nutrition
University of Minnesota Microbiota Therapeutics Program
Center for Immunology
BioTechnology Institute
Cancer Center
University of Minnesota
Minneapolis, Minnesota

Joann Kwah, MD, FACG
Assistant Professor of Medicine
Division of Gastroenterology
NYU Langone Medical Center
New York, New York

Neena Malik, MD, MSc
Gastroenterology Fellow
Division of Gastroenterology and Hepatology
Albert Einstein College of Medicine
Montefiore Medical Center
Bronx, New York

Paul Moayyedi, MD, PhD, MPH
Audrey Campbell Chair of Ulcerative Colitis Research
Farncombe Family Digestive Health Institute
McMaster University
Hamilton, Ontario, Canada

Benjamin H. Mullish, MB, BChir, MRCP, PhD
Clinical Lecturer
Division of Digestive Diseases
Department of Metabolism, Digestion and Reproduction
Faculty of Medicine
Imperial College London
London, United Kingdom

Sára Nemes, BA
Student
Indiana University School of Medicine
Indianapolis, Indiana

Majdi Osman, MD, MPH
Chief Medical Officer
OpenBiome
Cambridge, Massachusetts

Pratik Panchal, MD, MPH
Clinical Research Scientist
OpenBiome
Cambridge, Massachusetts

Abbas Rupawala, MD
Assistant Professor of Medicine
Warren Alpert Medical School of Brown University
Co-Director
Inflammatory Bowel Disease Center, Brown Medicine
Brown Physicians, Incorporated
Providence, Rhode Island

Lindsey Russell, MD, MSc
Gastroenterology Fellow
McMaster University
Hamilton, Ontario, Canada

Christopher Saddler, MD
Assistant Professor
Division of Infectious Disease
Department of Medicine
School of Medicine and Public Health
University of Wisconsin–Madison
Madison, Wisconsin

Nasia Safdar, MD, PhD
Professor
Division of Infectious Disease
Department of Medicine
School of Medicine and Public Health
University of Wisconsin–Madison
William S. Middleton Veterans Affairs Medical Center
Madison, Wisconsin

Neil Stollman, MD, FACP, FACG, AGAF
Associate Clinical Professor of Medicine
University of California San Francisco
San Francisco, California
Chief
Division of Gastroenterology
Alta Bates Summit Medical Center
Director of Research
East Bay Center for Digestive Health
Oakland, California

1

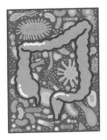

Introduction

*Jessica R. Allegretti, MD, MPH and
Zain Kassam, MD, MPH*

Mrs. Smith is an 82-year-old British woman who loosely resembles the Queen. She loves rose gardening and her grandchildren more than anything else in the world. Today, she is teary-eyed in clinic having suffered with *Clostridioides difficile* infection (CDI) for longer than she can remember. Most recently, she's been tied to the toilet for the past week and nearly fell rushing to the bathroom for her ninth watery bowel movement of the day. Five courses of antibiotics have failed to cure her CDI, and the symptoms seem to come back each time with more vengeance. Her grandson sent her an article on fecal transplants, and she wonders if this might be right for her.

Allegretti JR, Kassam Z, eds. *The 6 Ds of Fecal
Microbiota Transplantation: A Primer From
Decision to Discharge and Beyond* (pp 1-6).
© 2021 SLACK Incorporated.

Clinically, this scenario is strikingly common. The exponential rise of scientific literature and wide popular media coverage of both the microbiome and fecal microbiota transplantation (FMT) have ushered in the potential of the microbiome revolution in medicine. The elegant hypothesis that a patient's disease is a result of an abnormal microbiome, or dysbiosis, and if one restores the microbiome to homeostasis by FMT from a healthy donor it may treat, or even cure, a disease has captured the imagination of scientists, clinicians, and patients.

FMT is the first success story of a broader class of exciting microbiome therapeutics. A systematic review and meta-analysis of randomized clinical trials for FMT in recurrent *C. difficile* infection (rCDI) has reported a number needed to treat (NNT) of 3,[1] meaning a clinician needs to treat 3 rCDI patients with FMT to prevent rCDI in a single patient. By comparison, the NNT for aspirin following ST-elevation myocardial infarction to prevent a single death is 42.[2] Despite a lack of large, well-designed, placebo-controlled trials, the striking effect size for FMT and paucity of effective treatments for rCDI have led to its recommendation in both US and European CDI clinical practice guidelines.[3,4] Although data on FMT and microbiome therapeutics are continuing to emerge, this novel therapeutic is here to stay.

That said, the name *fecal microbiota transplantation* may not be here to stay. Many feel the term is not medically accurate, because the intervention transfers intestinal microbiota that engraft into a recipient, as opposed to transplanting feces, or stool, a complex substrate.[5] Additionally, the term may not be patient-centric and may dissuade patients who perceive FMT as the direct transfer of whole feces. Accordingly, the term *intestinal microbiota transplantation* and variations such as *intestinal microbiota transfer* or *intestinal microbiome therapy* have been proposed. As with many novel therapies, medical nomenclature changes; however, for the purpose of this book, we will continue to refer to the intervention as fecal microbiota transplantation or FMT.

Despite an evolving nomenclature, there is a major need for clinician-orientated education about FMT given the field is in its infancy. Practical FMT workshops or a dedicated clinical FMT fellowship is needed; however, currently these do not exist. So, how do medical trainees, practicing physicians, nurses, and allied health care members learn about the real-world aspects of FMT? That is the purpose of this book, *The 6 Ds of Fecal Microbiota Transplantation: A Primer From Decision to Discharge and Beyond*. This book aims to provide you with the practical tools and a simple clinical framework to understand FMT and administer end-to-end comprehensive FMT care. This book emphasizes practical pearls and checklists developed by leading world experts who have collectively cared for thousands of patients suffering from rCDI who have ultimately benefited from FMT. Given the popular media attention, patients often have questions about this novel therapy, and this book has practical responses to the most frequently asked questions.

Given the field of the microbiome is relatively new to clinicians, in Chapter 2, we review the nuts and bolts of the microbiome. What is it? How do you assess the microbiome? Why does it matter? Building on the new field of the microbiome, in Chapter 3 we revisit the history of the FMT, because to move forward, we must understand the past. When was FMT first described? How has it evolved?

From there, we introduce a simple practical framework for FMT: the 6 Ds.

1. *Decision*: Who is the right CDI patient to receive FMT? What clinical questions should you ask patients in your FMT clinical assessment?

2. *Donor*: How do you select a donor for FMT? How do you screen a donor?

3. *Discussion*: Navigating the risks, benefits, and alternatives in the informed consent process for FMT. What are the short-term risks? What are the long-term risks?

4. *Delivery*: What is the best delivery method for FMT? Should I use a colonoscopy, enema, or capsules?

5. *Discharge*: What is the ideal post-FMT care? How should I counsel my patients following FMT?

This pragmatic framework will provide clinicians with the real-world knowledge to administer FMT and navigate nuanced clinical cases of rCDI.

6. *Discovery*: We move beyond CDI and highlight the most promising clinical conditions in which FMT has been explored, from other gastrointestinal diseases, like irritable bowel syndrome and inflammatory bowel disease, to infectious conditions, such as enteric antibiotic-resistant bacteria, to liver and metabolic diseases and even neurological conditions. Overall, ongoing basic science and translational and clinical research are promising, and the search for the next condition to respond to microbiome therapies is underway.

As you navigate this book, you will learn the tips and tricks needed to counsel and manage patients like Mrs. Smith. And with time and care, you can provide her with the treatment she needs to break the cycle of CDI and return to her life as a rose gardener and grandmother.

References

1. Moayyedi P, Yuan Y, Baharith H, Ford AC. Faecal microbiota transplantation for *Clostridium difficile*-associated diarrhoea: a systematic review of randomised controlled trials. *Med J Aust*. 2017;207(4):166-172.
2. Randomized trial of intravenous streptokinase, oral aspirin, both, or neither among 17187 cases of suspected acute myocardial infarction: ISIS-2. ISIS-2 (Second International Study of Infarct Survival) Collaborative Group. *Lancet*. 1988;2(8607):349-360.
3. McDonald LC, Gerding DN, Johnson S, et al. Clinical practice guidelines for *Clostridium difficile* infection in adults and children: 2017 update by the Infectious Diseases Society of America (IDSA) and Society for Healthcare Epidemiology of America (SHEA). *Clin Infect Dis*. 2018;66(7):e1-e48.
4. Debast SB, Bauer MP, Kuijper EJ; European Society of Clinical Microbiology and Infectious Diseases. European Society of Clinical Microbiology and Infectious Diseases: update of the treatment guidance document for *Clostridium difficile* infection. *Clin Microbiol Infect*. 2014;20(suppl 2):1-26.
5. Khoruts A, Brandt LJ. Fecal microbiota transplant: a rose by any other name. *Am J Gastroenterol*. 2019;114(7):1176.

Abbreviations

AGA	American Gastroenterological Association
ARB	antibiotic-resistant bacteria
ASD	autism spectrum disorder
BMI	body mass index
BSS	Bristol stool score
CD	Crohn's disease
CDC	Centers for Disease Control and Prevention
CDI	*Clostridioides difficile* infection
CMV	cytomegalovirus
COVID-19	coronavirus disease 2019
CRE	carbapenem-resistant *Enterobacteriaceae*
DIY	do-it-yourself
EBV	Epstein-Barr virus
EMA	European Medicines Agency
EPEC	enteropathogenic *Escherichia coli*

ESBL	extended-spectrum beta-lactamase
FAQs	frequently asked questions
FDA	US Food and Drug Administration
FMT	fecal microbiota transplantation
GDH	glutamate dehydrogenase
GI	gastrointestinal
GMP	Good Manufacturing Practice
GvHD	graft vs host disease
IBD	inflammatory bowel disease
IBS	irritable bowel syndrome
IBS-C	constipation-predominant irritable bowel syndrome
IBS-D	diarrhea-predominant irritable bowel syndrome
IBS-M	mixed irritable bowel syndrome
ICI	immune checkpoint inhibitor
ICU	intensive care unit
IDSA	Infectious Diseases Society of America
IgG	immunoglobulin G
IND	Investigational New Drug
IPAA	ileal pouch–anal anastomosis
MRSA	methicillin-resistant *Staphylococcus aureus*
NAFLD	nonalcoholic fatty liver disease
NASH	nonalcoholic steatohepatitis
NGT	nasogastric tube
NNT	number needed to treat
OHE	overt hepatic encephalopathy
OR	odds ratio
PCR	polymerase chain reaction
PD	pharmacodynamic

PDAI	Pouchitis Disease Activity Index
PK	pharmacokinetic
PSC	primary sclerosing cholangitis
rCDI	recurrent *Clostridioides difficile* infection
rRNA	ribosomal RNA
RYGB	Roux-en-Y gastric bypass
SARS-CoV-2	severe acute respiratory syndrome coronavirus 2
SCFA	short-chain fatty acid
SIBO	small intestinal bacterial overgrowth
SOC	standard-of-care
SOT	solid organ transplant
STEC	Shiga toxin–producing *Escherichia coli*
toxin EIA	toxin enzyme immunoassay
UC	ulcerative colitis
UTI	urinary tract infection
VRE	vancomycin-resistant *Enterococcus*

2

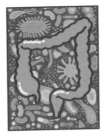

Microbiome 101

Suzanne Devkota, PhD

The gastrointestinal (GI) tract is a highly complex organ governed by tightly coordinated physiological processes that, at the same time, interact with a dense and diverse microbial population that both relies on us and exists independently of us. This gut microbiome is a critical player in our health from the moment we are born throughout life, and its reach extends far beyond our gut, affecting processes as distant as the brain. However, the direct effect of microbial colonization on gut development and physiology, and on conferring a competent mucosal immune system, has been demonstrated, and now established in the literature. Therefore, a deep understanding of external factors that affect colonization, such as diet, antibiotics, and exposure

Allegretti JR, Kassam Z, eds. *The 6 Ds of Fecal Microbiota Transplantation: A Primer From Decision to Discharge and Beyond* (pp 7-18).
© 2021 SLACK Incorporated.

to pathogens, is of critical importance as microbial-based therapies become mainstream. This chapter provides a practical overview of the microbiome for clinicians.

What Is the Microbiome?

The human body is colonized by bacteria, archaea, fungi, viruses, and protozoa that numerically equal or slightly outnumber our own human cells (Table 2-1). However, on a genomic level, these micro-organisms house an order of magnitude more genes than our own. And these genes, minute to minute, day to day, and over their lifespan, interact intimately with our human cells, especially in the gut, where the density of microbiota is the highest. These collections of microbes are called the *microbiota*, and their genes are called the *microbiome*. However, today, it is common for the term microbiome to be an all-encompassing term to refer to the body of organisms themselves, and often the bacterial fraction. Additional terms, such as *mycobiome* and *fungome*, referring to the fungal fraction, and *virome*, referring to the viral/phage fraction, are emerging to distinguish the study of these microbial compartments as distinct from the bacterial microbiome, despite the fact that the term microbiome technically refers to all of these microorganisms. However, it is indeed the bacterial component of the microbiome that outnumbers all the other life forms in the human gut, excluding bacteriophage, which are the most abundant but cannot survive independently. Although our understanding of the functions of these individual components continues to grow, what we do know is that the gut microbiome interacts closely with the immune, endocrine, and nervous systems. Therefore, changes in an individual's gut microbiome composition, that are a departure from their natural homeostasis, are correlated with an array of diseases and disorders, including inflammatory bowel diseases, Parkinson's disease, and cancer (Practical Pearl 2-1).[1-3]

Table 2-1. Simplified Framework of the Components of the Microbiome		
Classification	**Description**	**Comments**
Bacteria	Unicellular prokaryotic organisms that constitute the largest biomass of the human microbiome.	There are typical gut bacteria that are associated with health (e.g. *Faecalibacterium prausnitzii*) and pathogenic bacteria (e.g. *Mycobacterium tuberculosis*) which can lead to disease.
Archaea	Unicellular prokaryotic organisms similar to bacteria but without peptidoglycans.	The role of archaea in health and disease is emerging; *Methanobrevibacter smithii*, a key methane-producing organism, is associated with irritable bowel syndrome.
Fungi (fungome or mycobiome)	Multicellular eukaryotic organisms; complex microbe with growth and vegetative states.	May be harnessed for benefit in therapeutics (eg, *Saccharomyces boulardii*) or cause disease (eg, *Candida auris*).
Virus (virome)	Microorganism that requires a living cell to replicate; includes bacteriophage (target bacterial cells) and eukaryotic viruses (target human cells).	Bacteriophage therapy is being developed therapeutically to shape the microbiome and/or treat pathologic bacteria.
Protozoa/ helminths	Typically associated with sanitization conditions; however, emerging data suggest some protozoa are natural members of the gut microbiome.	Understudied component of the gut microbiome; some protozoa may be pathogenic, whereas diversity of protozoa have been linked to health. Similarly, helminthic therapy has been studied for inducing protective immune response in some people.

Practical Pearl 2-1

What Is Alpha Versus Beta Diversity?

When reviewing microbiome data and analysis, the most common findings reported are alpha and beta diversity, but what does this mean, and how are they measured?

Alpha Diversity
- The average number of different species within a sample.
- Common measure: Shannon diversity index; measures species evenness (eg, similar abundance or do some species dominate?); a higher Shannon diversity index value is more diverse than a lower value.

Beta Diversity
- Measures the differences between 2 samples.
- Common measure: Bray-Curtis dissimilarity; measures difference based on abundance (value between 0 and 1); a value of 0 means that both samples share the exact same species at the same abundance, whereas a value of 1 means that the 2 samples have a completely different species abundance.

Note: Although these are the most common ways to characterize microbiome diversity, newer and complementary methods are being developed.

Illustrative Example
Imagine the circles below are 2 stool samples, and the shapes represent different bacteria species. The conceptual alpha diversity of sample A and B is 3 (3 different species). The conceptual beta diversity of samples A and B is 2, because there are 2 distinct species between them.

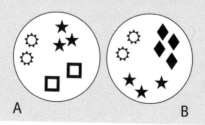

A   B

Historical Origins of Gut Microbiome Research

The field of the gut microbiome is relatively new. Its emergence as a scientific discipline became mainstream around 2005, when the cost of sequencing microbial genomes was significantly reduced. As data from the studies that followed emerged, discussion of manipulating the gut microbiome as a treatment modality in health care became a widespread part of the conversation, particularly in gastroenterology clinics. However, the microbiome field did not emerge spontaneously. It was a thoughtful evolution over time, rooted in fundamental discoveries in bacteriology and microbiology, the history of which provides a fascinating lens through which to appreciate the challenges and opportunities in modern-day microbiome medicine, particularly as it pertains to fecal microbiota transplantation (FMT).

In the early 1800s, disease was largely attributed to metaphysical factors, such as evil spirits, curses, or punishment for wrongdoings.[4] Early observations by Redi, Virchow, and Pasteur of sterile laboratory conditions disproved the theory of spontaneous generation, which was the accepted view at the time and stated that life erupted from nonliving material. Pasteur later discovered that fermentative processes were not caused by air, but rather by the yeast in the air. These observations were the beginnings of the germ theory of disease, which suggested that environmental microorganisms were the source of most diseases.[5,6]

Two subsequent seminal discoveries bridged the gap between environmental bacteriology and human disease. In 1876, Robert Koch, a German physician, proved that a single bacterium could directly cause a disease. He was asked to investigate why humans and livestock were mysteriously dying across Europe, and he discovered rod-shaped structures in the blood. Through a series of sophisticated experiments isolating these structures from blood and reintroducing them into healthy animals, he determined these structures were living bacteria, which he named *Bacillus anthracis*—or anthrax.[7] The experiments he conducted to identify anthrax led to the series of scientific principles known as Koch's postulates, which one uses to determine whether a particular bacterium is responsible for disease. These postulates have been slightly modified over time; however, they are still an accepted set of experiments for determining a bacterium's role in disease.[8] Yet, it was not until Theodor Escherich's 1885 discovery of the now-named *Escherichia coli,* isolated from the colons of healthy children, that evidence for gut-resident bacteria emerged. He determined that some of the *E. coli* strains were benign, whereas others were responsible for infant gastroenteritis. This was the first description of native gut microbiota, and also of strain variation of a bacterium in different contexts and individuals—a concept heavily investigated in the microbiome field today.[9-11]

The nearly 100 years that followed was an era of infectious disease control and vaccine development. These important efforts curtailed diseases that once killed by the thousands. This period was followed by a new era, led by Carl Woese and George Fox, that redefined the tree of life based on genetic signature rather than visual observations of morphology.[12] In their landmark paper, arguably one of the most influential microbiology publications to date, Woese and Fox showed that the ribosomal RNA (rRNA) of all living things organized all creatures into 3 categories: archaea, bacteria, and eukarya. The bacterial RNA signature was the 16S rRNA, and subsequent work by Norman Pace, Stanley Falkow, and David Relman applied the discovery of the 16S rRNA to show it could be reliably used to identify difficult-to-grow bacteria among mixed cellular communities[13] and that these tools could be applied to the identification of bacteria in humans.[14] With this, the genomic revolution of microbiology had begun, spawning the field of the modern-day microbiome (Table 2-2).

Microbiome Colonization in the Gut and Host Defenses

The gut harbors the densest community of microbes in the body, and the density of these microbes varies along the length of the GI tract (Figure 2-1), with the colon harboring the most numerous and diverse population. However, nothing happens by chance in the microbial ecology of the gut. The bacteria that colonize each segment of the GI tract are there because they have the ability to optimally survive in that particular niche amongst the daily chaos we subject them to at each meal, and in turn they serve a specialized function for the host. However, it is always a matter of survival of the fittest bacteria, with external and internal selection pressures creating a continually evolved community. For example, it was previously believed that the high acidity of the stomach prevented bacterial colonization, and therefore the stomach was essentially sterile. However, the stomach actually harbors a diverse, albeit not numerically large, community of commensal bacteria ranging from 10 to 100 bacteria/gram.[15] This diversity is dramatically reduced if *Helicobacter pylori* is present. *H. pylori* is uniquely adapted to the stomach environment such that it can outcompete all the other organisms and overgrow. It is the same

Table 2-2. Analysis Techniques for Characterizing Microbiota

Technique	Description	Comments
Cultivation	Isolation of living microorganisms from tissue, body fluids, or stool for in vitro testing or whole genome sequencing.	Inexpensive but labor intensive; allows for testing of antibiotic susceptibility and other functional properties of live microorganisms in real time.
16S rRNA sequencing	Targets the highly conserved 16S rRNA gene; compared with reference database of known bacteria to enable classification of the bacterial community.	Cost-effective technique that generates community composition and enables genus-level and, occasionally, species-level resolution.
Shotgun sequencing	Shotgun approach that generates entire genome; permits exploration of functional capacity with pathway prediction; captures bacteria, viruses, fungi, and host.	Costly and computationally intense technique that generates a deeper characterization and enables species- and subspecies-level resolution.
Metatranscriptomics	RNA sequencing that characterizes gene expression.	Highly expressed genes are most likely to be detected; requires immediate preservation or processing.
Metaproteomics	Mass spectrometry approach that characterizes protein expression.	Detects dominant proteins expressed; requires immediate preservation or processing.
Metabolomics	Mass spectrometry approach that characterizes metabolic capacity.	Targeted or untargeted approach that semiquantitatively detects metabolites; requires immediate preservation or processing.

Adapted from Allaband et al.[16]

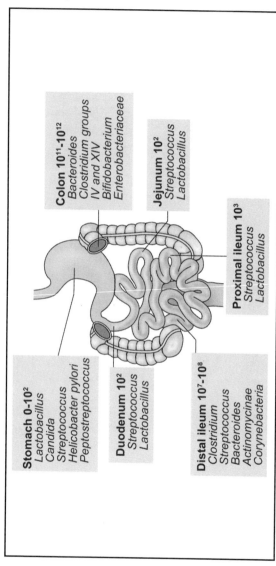

Figure 2-1. Select microbiome density by anatomical region in gastrointestinal tract.[17,18]

Colon 10¹¹-10¹²
Bacteroides
Clostridium groups
IV and XIV
Bifidobacterium
Enterobacteriaceae

Jejunum 10²
Streptococcus
Lactobacillus

Proximal ileum 10³
Streptococcus
Lactobacillus

Stomach 0-10²
Lactobacillus
Candida
Streptococcus
Helicobacter pylori
Peptostreptococcus

Duodenum 10²
Streptococcus
Lactobacillus

Distal ileum 10⁷-10⁸
Clostridium
Streptococcus
Bacteroides
Actinomycinae
Corynebacteria

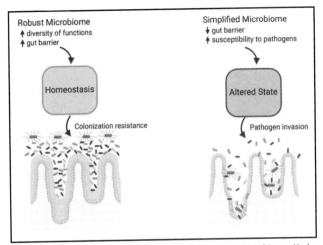

Figure 2-2. Pathogens thrive in the absence of a robust microbiome. Under homeostatic conditions (left), both the abundance and diversity of the gut microbiota confer a diversity of functions, including stimulating mucus production and niche occupation—all forms of barrier protections. However, when there is a disturbance of homeostasis (right) through chronic antibiotic use, the simplified microbiota can no longer provide the defensive barrier, allowing pathogens to invade.

phenomenon that governs *Clostridioides difficile* infection. When the commensal gut community is suppressed by antibiotics, *C. difficile* thrives. The colonization resistance that is often conferred by having a robust and diverse microbiome is no longer there, leaving an array of available niches exposed. Once *C. difficile* takes root and thrives, it can be very difficult to eradicate completely through standard-of-care antibiotics, leading to recurrent infection. This is, in large part, why FMT has proven so effective. To restore a microbially barren colon, a thriving, diverse community of organisms enters the GI tract like a SWAT team, occupying the niches and eradicating the offenders (Figure 2-2).

However, the intestines, too, have evolved sophisticated physical and immune-mediated defense strategies to contain the gut microbiota in the lumen and to distinguish the native from the foreign organisms. This largely starts at birth, when the infant experiences its first major exposure to microbiota upon entering the world. There is a dynamic feedback loop whereby expanding density and diversity of the early-life gut is required to build intestinal defense strategies that limit their expansion and translocation. For example, development of the epithelial cell brush border and tight junctions between cells is the result of bacterial colonization, but at the same time evolved to keep the microbiota sequestered. Other physical strategies include the continual cycle of crypt-to-villus migration, followed by epithelial cell shedding, which attenuates microbial attachment, and controlled cell death, which restricts microbial persistence. Naturally, many pathogens, such as adherent invasive *E. coli*, *Campylobacter jejuni*, and *Salmonella typhimurium*, have, in turn, evolved strategies to evade and neutralize these pathways.[19] Pathogen recognition receptors, such as toll-like receptors embedded in the gut epithelium, are continually surveying the local environment. We have learned much about these from studies in germ-free mice, which are mice raised from birth without a microbiome. These mice have immature intestinal defense and immune pathways; however, following an FMT of normal microbiota, all of the characteristics mentioned previously begin to develop. With exposure, these toll-like receptors are tuned, promoting tolerance of commensal microbes and heightened response to foreign pathogens. However, as would be expected, certain pathogens have developed ways to hijack these systems to evade detection. Through this understanding of pathogen colonization and evasion strategies and the critical role of natural bacterial colonization in maturation of the gut and its immune system, it becomes vitally clear that maintenance of a diverse and abundant commensal gut microbiome is a central feature of intestinal health.

Summary

The gut microbiome, including all its bacteria, fungi, viruses, and protozoa, numerically equal the number of human cells we have in our body. This scale of colonization is required to fully mature our GI tract, which is both the largest immune and endocrine organ in our body and the most highly innervated. This confluence of signals that converge at the gut, with this dense mixture of microbial cells, leads to profound opportunities to enhance health and develop therapies for treatment of disease. However, this also leads to a tenuous relationship between host microbe and outside pathogens that often aim to seek refuge in the confines of the GI tract. Unbeknownst to pathogens, in the presence of the healthy and robust microbiota, their colonization is often short lived. However, in immunologically or microbially compromised patients, the gut's primary defenses are lost, providing fertile ground for persistence and replication. Therefore, microbiome therapies, such as FMT, that restore microbiota become of the utmost importance (Practical Pearl 2-2).

Practical Pearl 2-2

What to Do When a Patient Brings Their Microbiome Analysis to Clinic?

- There are several commercial companies that provide microbiome analysis to patients who provide a stool sample.
- Your patient may bring a microbiome report to your office visit to discuss the results.
- Currently, the quality and clinical relevance of these microbiome reports is unknown and clinical decisions should not be made based on this analysis.

References

1. Frank DN, St. Amand AL, Feldman RA, et al. Molecular-phylogenetic characterization of microbial community imbalances in human inflammatory bowel diseases. *Proc Natl Acad Sci USA.* 2007;104(34):13780-13785.

2. Kostic AD, Chun E, Robertson L, et al. Fusobacterium nucleatum potentiates intestinal tumorigenesis and modulates the tumor-immune microenvironment. *Cell Host Microbe.* 2013;14(2):207-215.

3. Sampson TR, Debelius JW, Thron T, et al. Gut microbiota regulate motor deficits and neuroinflammation in a model of Parkinson's disease. *Cell.* 2016;167(6):1469-1480.e12.

4. Murphy D. Concepts of disease and health. In: Zalta EN, ed. *The Stanford encyclopedia of philosophy.* Stanford, CA: Stanford University Metaphysics Research Lab. Revised March 18, 2020. Accessed September 24, 2020. https://plato.stanford.edu/entries/health-disease

5. Schwartz M. The life and works of Louis Pasteur. *J Appl Microbiol.* 2001;91(4):597-601.

6. Bastian HC. The germ-theory of disease: being a discussion of the relation of bacteria and allied organisms to virulent inflammations and specific contagious fevers. *Br Med J.* 1875;1(745):469-476.

7. Blevins SM, Bronze MS. Robert Koch and the "golden age" of bacteriology. *Int J Infect Dis.* 2010;14(9):e744-751.

8. Falkow S. Molecular Koch's postulates applied to microbial pathogenicity. *Rev Infect Dis.* 1988;10(suppl 2):S274-S276.

9. Greenblum S, Carr R, Borenstein E. Extensive strain-level copy-number variation across human gut microbiome species. *Cell.* 2015;160(4):583-594.

10. Vatanen T, Plichta DR, Somani J, et al. Genomic variation and strain-specific functional adaptation in the human gut microbiome during early life. *Nat Microbiol.* 2019;4(3):470-479.

11. Lloyd-Price J, Mahurkar A, Rahnavard G, et al. Strains, functions and dynamics in the expanded Human Microbiome Project. *Nature.* 2017;550(7674):61-66.

12. Woese CR, Fox GE. Phylogenetic structure of the prokaryotic domain: the primary kingdoms. *Proc Natl Acad Sci USA.* 1977;74(11):5088-5090.

13. Lane DJ, Pace B, Olsen GJ, et al. Rapid determination of 16S ribosomal RNA sequences for phylogenetic analyses. *Proc Natl Acad Sci USA.* 1985;82(20):6955-6959.

14. Relman DA, Schmidt TM, MacDermott RP, et al. Identification of the uncultured bacillus of Whipple's disease. *N Engl J Med.* 1992;327(5):293-301.

15. Bik EM, Eckburg PB, Gill SR, et al. Molecular analysis of the bacterial microbiota in the human stomach. *Proc Natl Acad Sci USA.* 2006;103(3):732-737.

16. Allaband C, McDonald D, Vázquez-Baeza Y, et al. Microbiome 101: studying, analyzing, and interpreting gut microbiome data for clinicians. Clin Gastroenterol Hepatol. 2019;17(2):218-230 and Lynch SV, Pedersen O. The human intestinal microbiome in health and disease. *N Engl J Med.* 2016;375(24):2369-2379.

17. Paliy O. Research interests. Paliy Lab. Updated June 12, 2020. Accessed December 15, 2020. http://www.wright.edu/~oleg.paliy/research.html

18. Vanderhoof J, Pauley-Hunter R. Small intestinal bacterial overgrowth. In: Guandalini S, Dhawan A, Branski D, eds. *Textbook of Pediatric Gastroenterology, Hepatology and Nutrition.* Springer; 2016:487-494.

19. Shawki A, McCole DF. Mechanisms of intestinal epithelial barrier dysfunction by adherent-invasive *Escherichia coli. Cell Mol Gastroenterol Hepatol.* 2017;3(1):41-50.

3

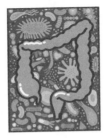

The History of Fecal Microbiota Transplantation

Joann Kwah, MD, FACG and
Lawrence J. Brandt, MD, MACG, AGAF, FASGE

Fecal microbiota transplantation (FMT) is the transfer of intestinal microbiota from a healthy donor to a recipient who has a certain disease with the intention of treating that disease.[1] Today, this concept is based on the knowledge that certain diseases are associated with an altered intestinal microbiome and the observation that restoration of a balanced, healthy intestinal microbiome may result in cure (eg, *Clostridioides difficile* infection [CDI]) or improvement of disease (eg, inflammatory bowel disease [IBD] or irritable bowel syndrome). The use of feces to treat a variety of ailments goes back more than 1000 years, but only recently has it gained recognition in humans as

Allegretti JR, Kassam Z, eds. *The 6 Ds of Fecal Microbiota Transplantation: A Primer From Decision to Discharge and Beyond* (pp 19-26).
© 2021 SLACK Incorporated.

a potential treatment for gastrointestinal (GI) diseases and, perhaps, for some non-GI diseases as well. This chapter reviews the history and evolution of FMT.

Early Use of Fecal Microbiota Transplantation

The use of FMT dates back to fourth century China, when Ge Hong described the use of human fecal suspension given by mouth for the treatment of food poisoning or severe diarrhea.[2] In the 16th century, Li Shizhen described oral administration of fermented fecal solution, fresh fecal suspension, dry feces, or infant feces for the treatment of severe diarrhea, fever, pain, vomiting, and constipation.[2] The fermented fecal solution was referred to as *yellow soup* to make it a more palatable nostrum. In the 17th century, cud (partially digested food from the first stomach of a ruminant) given orally and fecal suspensions given orally or by enema, termed *transfaunation*, were used in veterinary medicine to treat ruminants off feed with a variety of disorders and horses with chronic diarrhea.[3]

It was not until 1958, however, that Ben Eiseman, an American surgeon, wrote the first published report of fecal suspension used in Western medicine: a case series of 4 patients precariously ill with pseudomembranous enterocolitis caused by *Micrococcus pyogenes* and treated with fecal enemas. The stool donors used were surgical residents caring for the patients. The author notes dramatic improvement just hours after its administration.[4]

Nonetheless, FMT remained a largely forgotten therapy until 1983, when Schwan et al[5] reported the first case of FMT given by enema to treat CDI. Up until 1989, retention enemas had been the most common technique for FMT. In 1991, Aas et al[6] used a nasogastric tube as the route of administration. In 1998, Lund-Tønnesen administered stool via gastroscopy and colonoscopy.[7] In 2000, a case report by Persky and Brandt[8] described an older woman with CDI not responding to standard therapy who was symptomatically cured within several hours by one infusion of a saline suspension of her husband's stool administered colonoscopically by infusion. The material was infused in 10- to 20-mL increments every 10 cm throughout the colon upon withdrawal. This report served to raise awareness of this therapy for recurrent CDI (rCDI).

Fecal Microbiota Transplantation in the 21st Century

Silverman et al[9] detailed the self-administration of FMT by enema in 2010 with donors screened by physicians, which resulted in the wider use of FMT. The use of FMT capsules were first reported by Louie et al,[10] who administered 24 to 34 capsules to 27 patients with CDI and achieved a 100% cure rate. Additionally, Hamilton et al[11] in 2012 reported that frozen FMT was just as effective as fresh FMT, which served to show that stool samples could be processed at a Good Manufacturing Practice (GMP) facility and shipped safely without loss of therapeutic effect over long distances, thus greatly increasing availability of FMT. It has since been noted by others that FMT administered via processed frozen fecal suspensions has efficacy rates similar to those of FMT performed using fresh stool.[12] The possibility of widespread distribution from a central facility has been proven by a large US stool bank (OpenBiome, Cambridge, MA), which supports access to FMT. As of October 2019, the stool bank has reported shipping more than 50,000 FMT treatments to physicians in 50 states and 7 countries (Practical Pearl 3-1).[13]

As the delivery of FMT evolves from fresh fecal suspensions to the use of frozen material processed under GMP best practices, the content of the product is also changing. Historically, Tvede and Rask-Madsen[14] demonstrated the effectiveness of a 10-bacterial strain combination to successfully treat 5 patients with rCDI. The authors concluded that the 3 species in this combination contributing to remission belonged to the *Bacteroides* genus (*B. ovatus*, *B. thetaiotaomicron*, and *B. vulgatus*). Graham et al[15] subsequently confirmed the role of *Bacteroides* species, curing 1 patient with rCDI with the same 3 species of *Bacteroides*. There is now a sector within the biotechnology industry devoted to microbiome therapeutics, where companies such as Finch Therapeutics Group Inc, Seres Therapeutics Inc, and Rebiotix Inc are developing technologies to restore a healthy composition of microbes. Clinical trials are ongoing with these microbiome therapies for diseases including CDI and IBD (Table 3-1).

Practical Pearl 3-1

Is All Fecal Microbiota Transplantation the Same?

- Over time, the level of manufacturing requirements that constitutes a safe FMT have increased.
- First-generation FMT, described by Eiseman et al[4] as a "fecal enema" without any manipulation, filtering, or donor screening, is no longer the current standard.
- In comparison, current-generation FMT products from stool banks have rigorous donor screening and apply significant processing under GMP manufacturing practice; however, patients performing do-it-yourself FMT or individual clinicians attempting FMT may not adhere to the same screening or manufacturing standards.
- Accordingly, there is ongoing conflation of the term FMT in the field, and it is important for clinicians to recognize that donor screening, manufacturing processing, cryoprotectant, formulation, delivery, and dose have an impact on both the safety and efficacy outcomes.
- Given the variability in donor material procurement and processing of FMT, safety and efficacy from one FMT product may not have the same results as another, and clinicians must be mindful to apply best practices in evidence-based medicine.

Table 3-1. History of Nomenclature for Transplantation of Fecal Microbiota

Yellow soup	Fecal infusion
Bacteriotherapy	Stool transfer
Fecal therapy	Stool transplant
Fecal transplant	Intestinal microbiome restoration
Fecal microbiota transplant	Intestinal microbiota transplantation (variations: intestinal microbiota transfer, intestinal microbiome therapy)

US Food and Drug Administration Guidance for Fecal Microbiota Transplantation

One critical issue in the midst of the evolution and growth of FMT is guidance for its utilization by the practicing gastroenterologist, as well as oversight and regulation provided by the FDA. In 2010, members of various specialty societies with an interest in FMT formed a working group for the purpose of creating a network of practitioners who could offer FMT to patients with CDI and developing an early protocol whereby FMT could be performed as safely as possible.[16] A consensus on FMT use for CDI included recurrent or relapsing infection (> 3 episodes), moderate CDI not responding to standard therapy for at least 1 week, or severe CDI with no response to standard therapy after 48 hours.[16] In 2013, the American College of Gastroenterology established treatment guidelines for CDI and recommended FMT as a therapeutic alternative for rCDI failing to respond to a pulsed/tapered regimen of vancomycin.[17] These recommendations were based on compelling, but observational, clinical experience describing the overwhelming success of FMT for this infection, but there was a lack of randomized controlled trials to support its efficacy and place in the treatment paradigm.

Finally, the first randomized clinical trial using FMT in which duodenal infusion of donor feces was given to patients with rCDI following standard-of-care antibiotics and showed significant efficacy in resolving symptoms compared with antibiotics alone, with an overall cure rate in the FMT group of 94% was published in the Netherlands in 2013.[18] Several other randomized clinical trials followed that were successful, but in May 2013, the FDA announced that stool would be considered a biologic agent/drug because it was being used with therapeutic intent and, therefore, FMT would be regulated like an investigational drug. This would require physicians and scientists to file an Investigational New Drug (IND) application before conducting an FMT. Because the impact of these regulations would limit patient access to FMT, patients, physicians, and medical professional societies rallied to advocate for an alternative approach.

In July 2013, the FDA issued a guidance statement that it would exercise enforcement discretion to allow physicians the ability to provide FMT for patients with CDI not responsive to standard therapies without an IND application, as long as informed consent was obtained and the patient was told that use of FMT was investigational. In March 2016, the FDA released a new draft guidance statement that narrowed the scope of enforcement discretion and would require an IND if material was being obtained from a stool bank, although an IND was not needed if physicians and hospitals collected and screened donor stool for FMT. This new draft guidance heightened concerns regarding access to FMT for patients suffering with rCDI but also highlighted the continuing need for discussions on how FMT should be regulated. This draft guidance, as of October 2020, has not been enacted, and stool banks continue to operate without an IND requirement for CDI not responsive to standard therapy. Though, in light of the global health pandemic of COVID-19 and the potential risk of SARS-CoV-2 transmission via FMT, the FDA instituted additional protections for any investigational use of FMT, including no clinical use of FMT products that were donated or manufactured on or after December 1, 2019 unless tested for SARS-CoV-2 virus. Additionally, the FDA have required that the informed consent process be updated to include the risk of SARS-CoV-2 via FMT. It has been suggested that FMT from stool banks be regulated in same manner as human cell-tissue establishment with additional oversight and "modified stool-based products" regulated as biological drugs.[19] Finally, the widespread availability of FMT has been suggested to hamper the ability of industry to recruit sufficient numbers of patients for clinical trials, which are, of course, placebo controlled. This issue is under active debate now, and the FDA's final determination on how FMT will be regulated is still pending at the time of writing.

Summary

FMT is a promising treatment that has evolved from early Chinese medicine to current next-generation microbiome therapies. It has served to focus our attention on the intestinal microbiome. The future looks to be very exciting as we learn how important the microbiome is—not only in causing disease but in maintaining health. Although the regulation of FMT by the FDA is still being refined, research is ongoing to help target our ability to more precisely treat disease in a standardized and safe fashion; long-term data collection on patients who have received FMT will be of great use to achieve this goal. The future is certain to reveal innovative ways to use microbiome therapies such as FMT for both GI and non-GI diseases and to revolutionize how we approach disease management.

References

1. Khoruts AJ, Brandt LJ. Fecal microbiota transplant: a rose by any other name. *Am J Gastroenterol.* 2019;114(7):1176.

2. Zhang F, Luo W, Shi Y, Fan Z, Ji G. Should we standardize the 1,700-year old fecal microbiota transplantation? *Am J Gastroenterol.* 2012;107(11):1755-1756.

3. Borody TJ, Warren EF, Leis SM, Surace R, Ashman O, Siarakas S. Bacteriotherapy using fecal flora: toying with human motions. *J Clin Gastroenterol.* 2004;38(6):475-483.

4. Eiseman B, Silen W, Bascom GS, Kauvar AJ. Fecal enema as an adjunct in the treatment of pseudomembranous enterocolitis. *Surgery.* 1958;44(5):854-859.

5. Schwan A, Sjölin S, Trottestam U, Aronsson B. Relapsing *Clostridium difficile* enterocolitis cured by rectal infusion of homologous faeces. *Lancet.* 1983;2(8354):845.

6. Aas J, Gessert CE, Bakken JS. Recurrent *Clostridium difficile* colitis case series involving 18 patients treated with donor stool administered via a nasogastric tube. *Clin Infect Dis.* 2003;36(5):580-585.

7. Lund-Tønnesen S, Berstad A, Schreiner A, Midtvedt T. *Clostridium difficile*–assosiert diare behandlet med homolog feces. *Tidsskr Nor Laegeforen.* 1998;118:1027-1030.

8. Persky S, Brandt LJ. Treatment of recurrent *Clostridium difficile*–associated diarrhea by administration of donated stool directly through a colonoscope. *Am J Gastroenterol.* 2000;95(11):3283-3285.

9. Silverman MS, Davis I, Pillai DR. Success of self-administered home fecal transplantation for chronic *Clostridium difficile* infection. *Clin Gastroenterol Hepatol.* 2010;8(5):471-473.

10. Louie T, Cannon K, O'Grady H, Wu K, Ward L. Fecal microbiome transplantation (FMT) via oral fecal microbial capsules for recurrent *Clostridium difficile* infection (rCDI). Abstract 89. Presented at: ID Week 2013; October 2-6, 2013; San Francisco, CA. Accessed June 10, 2020. https://idsa.confex.com/idsa/2013/webprogram/Paper41627.html

11. Hamilton MJ, Weingarden AR, Unno T, Khoruts A, Sadowsky MJ. High-throughput DNA sequence analysis reveals stable engraftment of gut microbiota following transplantation of previously frozen fecal bacteria. *Gut Microbes.* 2013;4(2):125-135.

12. Youngster I, Russell GH, Pindar C, Ziv-Baran T, Sauk J, Hohmann EL. Oral, capsulized, frozen fecal microbiota transplantation for relapsing *Clostridium difficile* infection. *JAMA.* 2014;312(17):1772-1778.

13. Onsite with OpenBiome. *Healio Gastroenterology.* January 17, 2017. Accessed September 24, 2020. https://www.healio.com/news/gastroenterology/20170112/onsite-with-openbiome

14. Tvede M, Rask-Madsen J. Bacteriotherapy for chronic relapsing *Clostridium difficile* diarrhoea in six patients. *Lancet.* 1989;1(8648):1156-1160.

15. Graham D, Attumi T, Opekun AR, et al. Triple *Bacteroides* fecal replacement therapy for relapsing *Clostridium difficile* diarrhea (fecal transplantation sans feces). *Am J Gastroenterol.* 2013;108(2):S170.

16. Bakken JS, Borody T, Brandt LJ, et al. Treating *Clostridium difficile* infection with fecal microbiota transplantation. *Clin Gastroenterol Hepatol.* 2011;9(12):1044-1049.

17. Surawicz CM, Brandt LJ, Binion DG, et al. Guidelines for diagnosis, treatment, and prevention of *Clostridium difficile* infections. *Am J Gastroenterol.* 2013;108(4):478-499.

18. van Nood E, Vrieze A, Nieuwdorp M, et al. Duodenal infusion of donor feces for recurrent *Clostridium difficile. N Engl J Med.* 2013;368(5):407-415.

19. Hoffmann D, Palumbo F, Ravel J, Roghmann MC, Rowthorn V, von Rosenvinge E. Improving regulation of microbiota transplants. *Science.* 2017;358(6369):1390-1391.

4

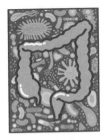

Decision

Which Patients With *Clostridioides difficile* Infection Are Appropriate for Fecal Microbiota Transplantation?

Abbas Rupawala, MD and Colleen R. Kelly, MD

Clostridioides difficile (previously *Clostridium difficile*) is an anaerobic gram-positive bacillus that has emerged as the most common cause of hospital-acquired infection in the past 2 decades. The incidence of recurrent *C. difficile* infection (rCDI) has nearly doubled since 2001, and multiply-recurrent infection has increased nearly 200% over the same period of time.[1] Factors including the increased use of antibiotics and their effect on gut microbiota and the emergence of more virulent strains have contributed to the higher occurrence of both health care–associated and community-acquired *C. difficile* infection (CDI) as well as more severe and fulminant cases. Although an altered gut microbiome

Allegretti JR, Kassam Z, eds. *The 6 Ds of Fecal Microbiota Transplantation: A Primer From Decision to Discharge and Beyond* (pp 27-41). © 2021 SLACK Incorporated.

is central to the pathophysiology of CDI, the standard treatment for primary and recurrent episodes remains antibiotics, often given as long, tapering courses, which control the infection but do little to restore the microbiome to a healthy, diverse state.

A number of small randomized clinical trials have reported high efficacy rates for fecal microbiota transplantation (FMT) following standard-of-care (SOC) antibiotics to prevent rCDI,[2] and FMT is increasingly being used in acute severe and fulminant disease.[3,4] In this chapter, we will review the relevant data supporting FMT for treatment of CDI as well as the clinical evaluation, diagnostic dilemmas, and decision making around administering FMT.

Recurrent
Clostridioides difficile Infection

The efficacy of FMT following SOC antibiotics for preventing rCDI has been well described in numerous case series and randomized clinical trials, with clinical cure rates reported from 68% to 100%. The first randomized clinical trial evaluating the efficacy of FMT in rCDI, in which FMT was administered by nasoduodenal infusion and showed statistically superior cure rates (81% for single administration) compared with vancomycin (31%), and the trial was stopped early by the institutional research board for benefit, was published in 2013.[5] Subsequently, other small randomized clinical trials in rCDI have largely replicated these results when comparing FMT following SOC antibiotics to other interventions, including autologous stool transplant as placebo,[6] vancomycin alone,[7] and fidaxomicin alone.[8] Efficacy has been reported as similar with fresh, frozen,[9] and lyophilized material,[10] and high success rates have been observed regardless of mode of FMT administration, including oral capsules (Table 4-1).[11]

Most investigators have defined rCDI as 3 or more episodes, although a number of trials have performed FMT after 2 episodes. Overall, the number needed to treat for FMT is 3 (95% confidence interval, 2-7) to prevent CDI recurrence following SOC antibiotics.[2] Although there is variation and a lack of consensus on the definition of rCDI, all CDI clinical practice guidelines recommend FMT for individuals who have suffered more than 3 CDI episodes (2 or more recurrences).[12-14]

Although CDI diagnosis may be obvious, such as in a patient presenting with profuse watery diarrhea and leukocytosis who responds clinically to oral vancomycin, some patients present with atypical symptoms, and relying heavily on results of polymerase chain reaction (PCR)–based stool testing may result in diagnostic errors. Studies from high-volume tertiary centers have reported alternative, non-CDI diagnoses in as many as 25% of patients referred for rCDI.[15,16] Highly sensitive molecular testing detects the presence of the toxin gene (may or may not be on), and if PCR-based stool tests are used in isolation, they may lead to a high false-positive rate for the diagnosis of CDI. In contrast to toxin enzyme immunoassays (toxin EIA) test directly for the presence of toxins and have a high specificity. Clinical guidelines recommend a 2-step algorithm with a highly sensitive test (PCR or glutamate dehydrogenase [GDH]) followed by a highly specific test (toxin EIA).

Rates of asymptomatic *C. difficile* colonization with a toxigenic strain are as high as 15% in heathy adults and may reach 50% in residents of long-term care facilities.[17] Patients who are colonized and have a non-CDI etiology of diarrheal symptoms may be incorrectly classified as CDI if only the results of a PCR assay are considered. Furthermore, post-infection irritable bowel syndrome (IBS) is common after CDI,[18] and these colonized patients with ongoing diarrheal symptoms may be treated unnecessarily with repeated courses of vancomycin or FMT (Figure 4-1).

Obtaining a detailed history around the CDI is important (Practical Pearls 4-1 and 4-2). Patients who are inappropriately tested for cure after resolution of diarrheal symptoms and found to be stool PCR positive should not be treated or considered for FMT. Atypical features, such as intermittent, nonprogressive symptoms and nonresponse to SOC antibiotics (eg, vancomycin), should raise concern that a patient's symptoms are not due to CDI. Patients who describe long duration of symptoms (months) prior to initial diagnosis are unlikely to be experiencing CDI as the source of those symptoms. In terms of laboratory investigations, because PCR-positive, toxin EIA–negative patients do not appear to experience complications or require treatment,[19] it is recommended to conduct a 2-step *C. difficile* testing algorithm instead of using a PCR-based stool test alone. Fecal calprotectin, a marker of gastrointestinal (GI) inflammation, is typically elevated in CDI and may also be helpful in distinguishing colonization from active infection. Specifically, a fecal calprotectin that is low or normal may suggest colonization as compared with a CDI episode.[20] In patients where the diagnosis of CDI is uncertain, workup may also include celiac serologies, *Giardia* testing, fecal fat stain, and colonoscopy with mucosal biopsies to exclude inflammatory bowel disease (IBD) and microscopic colitis.

Table 4-1. Summary of Prospective Randomized Clinical Trials of Fecal Microbiota Transplantation for *Clostridioides difficile* Infection

Author (Year)	Country	Sample Size	Population	Intervention
Trials Comparing Fecal Microbiota Transplantation With Standard-of-Care Antibiotics With or Without a Placebo				
van Nood et al (2013)[5]	Netherlands	42	CDI recurrence (> 2 episodes)	Short course of vancomycin followed by bowel lavage and FMT via nasoduodenal tube
Cammarota et al (2015)[7]	Italy	39	CDI recurrence (> 2 episodes)	Short course of vancomycin followed by bowel lavage and FMT via colonoscopy
Kelly et al (2016)[6]	United States	46	> 3 CDI recurrences (> 4 episodes)	Standard course of vancomycin followed by bowel lavage and FMT via colonoscopy
Hota et al (2017)[21]	Canada	30	> 2 CDI recurrences (> 3 episodes)	Standard course of vancomycin followed by FMT via enema
Hvas et al (2019)[8]	Denmark	64	CDI recurrence (> 2 episodes)	Short course of vancomycin followed by FMT via colonoscopy or nasojejunal tube

Table 4-1. Summary of Prospective Randomized Clinical Trials of Fecal Microbiota Transplantation for *Clostridioides difficile* Infection

Comparator	Outcome	Result
Trials Comparing Fecal Microbiota Transplantation With Standard-of-Care Antibiotics With or Without a Placebo		
Vancomycin (500 mg QID x 14 days) or vancomycin with bowel lavage	At week 10, absence of diarrhea or persistent diarrhea explicable by other causes with 3 consecutive negative *C. difficile* tests	FMT arm: 13/16 (81%) resolution ($P < 0.001$ for both comparisons) Vancomycin alone arm: 4/13 (31%) resolution Vancomycin with bowel lavage arm: 3/13 (23%)
Vancomycin (125 mg QID x 10 days) followed by 125 to 500 mg/day every 2 to 3 days for >3 weeks	At week 10, absence of diarrhea or persistent diarrhea explicable by other causes with 2 negative *C difficile* tests	FMT arm: 18/20 (90%) resolution ($P < 0.0001$) Vancomycin arm: 5/19 (26%) resolution
Standard course of vancomycin followed by sham FMT (placebo; autologous material)	At week 8, absence of diarrhea without need for CDI antibiotics	FMT arm: 20/22 (91%) resolution ($P = 0.042$) Placebo arm: 15/24 (63%) resolution
Vancomycin taper for 6 weeks	At day 120, no recurrence of CDI	FMT arm: 9/16 (66%) resolution ($P = $ NS) Vancomycin arm: 5/12 (42%)
Fidaxomicin (200 mg BID x 10 days) or vancomycin (125 mg QID x 10 days)	At week 8, clinical resolution and a negative *C difficile* test result without the need for rescue FMT or colectomy	FMT arm: 17/24 (71%) resolution ($P = 0.009$ FMT vs fidaxomicin; $P = 0.001$ FMT vs vancomycin) Fidaxomicin alone arm: 8/24 (33%) resolution Vancomycin alone arm: 3/16 (19%) resolution *(continued)*

Table 4-1 (continued). Summary of Prospective Randomized Clinical Trials of Fecal Microbiota Transplantation for *Clostridioides difficile* Infection

Author (Year)	Country	Sample Size	Population	Intervention
Trials Comparing Fecal Microbiota Transplantation Delivery Modalities				
Youngster et al (2014)[22]	United States	20	>2 CDI recurrences (>3 episodes of mild-moderate CDI with vancomycin failure) or CDI recurrence (>2 severe episodes resulting in hospitalization); SOC antibiotics discontinued at least 48 hours prior to procedure	Bowel lavage and FMT via colonoscopy; single dose of loperamide at time of procedure
Lee et al (2016)[9]	Canada	219	Refractory CDI or CDI recurrence; patients with only a single CDI recurrence (2 episodes) were not included unless the most recent episode became refractory to treatment; SOC antibiotics discontinued 24 to 48 hours prior to procedure	FMT (frozen) enema

Table 4-1. Summary of Prospective Randomized Clinical Trials of Fecal Microbiota Transplantation for *Clostridioides difficile* Infection

Comparator	Outcome	Result
Trials Comparing Fecal Microbiota Transplantation Delivery Modalities		
FMT via NGT; proton pump inhibitor administered for 48 hours prior to procedure	At week 8, absence of diarrhea without need for CDI antibiotics	FMT via colonoscopy arm: 8/10 (80%) resolution FMT via NGT arm: 6/10 (60%) resolution
FMT (fresh) enema	At week 13, absence of diarrhea without need for CDI antibiotics after receiving up to 2 FMTs	Single FMT via enema (frozen): 57/108 (53%) resolution Single FMT via enema (fresh): 56/111 (51%)

(continued)

Table 4-1 (continued). Summary of Prospective Randomized Clinical Trials of Fecal Microbiota Transplantation for *Clostridioides difficile* Infection

Author (Year)	Country	Sample Size	Population	Intervention
Trials Comparing Fecal Microbiota Transplantation Delivery Modalities				
Kao et al (2017)[11]	Canada	116	> 2 CDI recurrences (> 3 episodes)	Standard course of vancomycin followed by bowel lavage and FMT via capsules
Jiang et al (2017)[10]	United States	72	> 2 CDI recurrences (> 3 episodes); SOC antibiotics discontinued 48 hours prior to the procedure	Bowel lavage followed by FMT by colonoscopy (lyophilized)
Jiang et al (2018)[23]	United States	65	> 2 CDI recurrences (> 3 episodes; SOC antibiotics discontinued 48 hours prior to the procedure	Bowel lavage and loperamide followed by FMT capsules (lyophilized)

Abbreviations: NGT = nasogastric tube; QID = 4 times/day.

Table 4-1. Summary of Prospective Randomized Clinical Trials of Fecal Microbiota Transplantation for *Clostridioides difficile* Infection

Comparator	Outcome	Result
Trials Comparing Fecal Microbiota Transplantation Delivery Modalities		
Standard course of vancomycin followed by bowel lavage and FMT via colonoscopy	At week 12, absence of CDI	FMT via capsule: 51/53 (96%) resolution FMT via colonoscopy: 50/52 (96%) resolution
Bowel lavage followed by FMT by colonoscopy (frozen and fresh)	At 2 months, absence of CDI	FMT via colonoscopy (lyophilized): 16/23 (78%) resolution FMT via colonoscopy (frozen): 20/24 (83%) resolution FMT via colonoscopy (fresh): 25/25 (100%) resolution
Bowel lavage and loperamide followed FMT by enema	At 2 months, absence of CDI	FMT via capsules (lyophilized): 26/31 (84%) resolution FMT via enema: 30/34 (88%) resolution

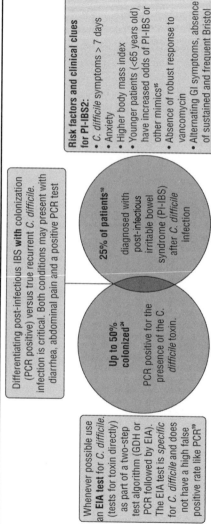

Figure 4-1. Clinical considerations in the diagnosis of C. difficile infection.[15,18,19,24]

Risk factors and clinical clues for PI-IBS2:
- *C. difficile* symptoms > 7 days
- Anxiety
- Higher body mass index
- Younger patients (<65 years old) have increased odds of PI-IBS or other mimics[15]
- Absence of robust response to vancomycin
- Alternating GI symptoms, absence of sustained and frequent Bristol stool score Type 6-7 stool

Differentiating post-infectious IBS **with** colonization (PCR positive) versus true recurrent *C. difficile* infection is critical. Both conditions may present with diarrhea, abdominal pain and a positive PCR test

25% of patients[18]

diagnosed with post-infectious irritable bowel syndrome (PI-IBS) after *C. difficile* infection

Irritable bowel syndrome (IBS) is a common functional gastrointestinal condition. PI-IBS is common among patients after *C. difficile*.

Up to 50% colonized[24]

PCR positive for the presence of the *C. difficile* toxin.

Stool that is PCR positive for the presence of the *C. difficile* toxin gene (not the toxin itself) often suggests **colonization.**

Whenever possible use an **EIA test** for *C. difficile* (tests for toxin directly) as part of a two-step test algorithm (GDH or PCR followed by EIA). The EIA test is *specific* for *C. difficile* and does not have a high false positive rate like PCR[19]

Practical Pearl 4-1

Assessing Eligibility for Fecal Microbiota Transplantation: CRAP Approach

Confirm True CDI
- Confirm laboratory test used to make diagnosis of CDI (eg, PCR alone vs 2-step testing [PCR or GDH with reflex to toxin EIA])
  - If PCR positive and toxin EIA negative, was patient on empiric CDI antibiotics at time of test?
- Confirm patient has responded to vancomycin or fidaxomicin.
- Conduct a detailed diarrhea assessment (eg, frequency, duration, Bristol stool score [BSS] type, pattern/trajectory, nocturnal symptoms, associated symptoms).
  - CDI tends to have > 3 non-bloody bowel movements/day (BSS 6-7) that progressively worsen without treatment.

Rule Out Mimics
- Conduct a detailed assessment to rule out alternative diagnoses, especially in younger patients (< 65 years) who are more likely to have a non-CDI diagnosis.
- Post-infection IBS
  - Often less frequent bowel movements, lower BSS, alternating/nonprogressive pattern, no nocturnal symptoms, commonly associated with bloating.
- New diagnosis of IBD or IBD flare
  - May have bloody diarrhea, extraintestinal manifestations of IBD, nocturnal symptoms.
- Other causes of diarrhea
  - Exclude celiac disease, bile salt diarrhea, microscopic colitis, etc.

Asses for Risk of FMT Failure
- IBD
- Immunosuppression
- Solid organ transplant
- Severe or fulminant CDI
- Ongoing systemic antibiotic use

Probe for Potential Complication Risks
- Significant immunosuppression (eg, absolute neutrophil count < 1000 /μL)
- Motility disorders (FMT via upper GI delivery)
- Dysphagia (FMT via capsule)

Practical Pearl 4-2

Beyond the CRAP Approach, What Additional Information Should You Gather During a Fecal Microbiota Transplantation Consult?

- ❑ Inciting antibiotics and indication for antibiotics
- ❑ CDI testing used for diagnosis of each episode (PCR alone vs 2-step with toxin EIA)
- ❑ Each previous CDI treatment course and clinical response to SOC treatments
- ❑ CDI-related hospitalizations
- ❑ CDI symptoms and severity (eg, diarrhea, abdominal pain, fever, fecal incontinence)
- ❑ Atypical features (eg, long symptom duration prior to initial diagnosis, nonresponse to vancomycin, intermittent/nonprogressive symptoms)
- ❑ Pre-CDI GI issues (eg, IBS, IBD, chronic diarrhea)
- ❑ Ongoing need for non-CDI antibiotics
- ❑ Planned surgery or other procedure that may require antibiotics in the near future
- ❑ Pregnant/planned pregnancy

This workup is particularly important in younger patients (< 65 years) who are at highest risk for an alternative diagnosis mimicking rCDI.[15,16]

FMT should not be offered to colonized patients or those who are experiencing post-infection IBS. Patients who have limited life expectancy (< 1 year) or who are likely to continue to require frequent courses of antibiotics are also poor candidates for FMT and should be considered for long-term suppressive vancomycin. In patients who are planning to have elective surgery, such as an orthopedic procedure, it makes sense to maintain oral vancomycin though the perioperative and early postoperative periods to prevent further recurrence and schedule the FMT once the patient has recovered. Patients residing in short-term rehabilitation facilities may continue to have antibiotic and *C. difficile* exposure, so continuing vancomycin and timing FMT to when the patient is nearing discharge or has been discharged home may reduce the probability of FMT failure. Although FMT capsules and FMT by colonoscopy are equally effective,[11] it is reasonable to perform FMT by the colonoscopic approach in rCDI patients who have not had a recent colonoscopy, to exclude comorbid IBD.[22]

Refractory
Clostridioides difficile Infection

There is not a standardized definition of refractory CDI, and the term is not described in current clinical guidelines, which categorize CDI as non-severe, severe, and fulminant.[14] To add to the confusion, the terms *recurrent* and *refractory* are often used interchangeably in the literature. In general, refractory CDI is most commonly used to describe patients with CDI who do not respond to SOC antibiotic treatment, although these patients often meet criteria for severe disease that is nonresponsive to SOC antibiotics. Two randomized clinical trials included such patients, one with failure to respond to treatment for 5 days, and another for 3 weeks. Outcomes of FMT in this patient group were comparable to rCDI.[9,13] Experts recommend FMT be considered in patients not responding to at least 1 week of SOC antibiotics (eg, vancomycin). Flexible sigmoidoscopy may be useful to confirm the diagnosis (eg, presence of pseudomembranes) and exclude other pathology, such as IBD, which may be driving ongoing symptoms.

Severe and Fulminant
Clostridioides difficile Infection

The 2017 Infectious Diseases Society of American guidelines define patients with severe CDI as those with leukocytosis (white blood cells $\geq 15,000$ cells/mm^3) or acute kidney injury with a serum creatinine of greater than 1.5 g/dL, and define fulminant CDI infection as being accompanied by hypotension or shock, ileus, or megacolon.[14] Other clinical CDI guidelines include end organ failure, intensive care unit (ICU) admission, mental status changes, lactic acidosis, and high fever as suggestive of severe or fulminant infection.[12] These factors help identify patients who are at high risk for colectomy or death. The past decade has seen an increase in cases of severe and fulminant CDI, which are the primary causes of increased mortality and morbidity of *C. difficile*, including prolonged hospital stay, ICU admission, malnutrition, and colectomy. These patients may be considered for FMT; however, data suggest the therapeutic strategy may be different (see Chapter 10.1.2: "The Role of Fecal Microbiota Transplantation in the Treatment of Severe and Fulminant *Clostridioides difficile* Infection").

Summary

Although previously considered a treatment of last resort, FMT with preceding *C. difficile* antibiotics has now become SOC in the prevention of rCDI. Patients should not be made to suffer months of recurrences and fail numerous, prolonged courses of antibiotics before being offered an FMT. Although questions remain around donor selection, screening methods, and ideal routes of administration, these should not deter physicians from implementing FMT into clinical practice.

References

1. Ma GK, Brensinger CM, Wu Q, Lewis JD. Increasing incidence of multiply recurrent *Clostridium difficile* infection in the United States: a cohort study. *Ann Intern Med.* 2017;167(3):152-158.

2. Moayyedi P, Yuan Y, Baharith H, Ford AC. Faecal microbiota transplantation for *Clostridium difficile*-associated diarrhoea: a systematic review of randomised controlled trials. *Med J Aust.* 2017;207(4):166-172.

3. Fischer M, Sipe B, Cheng YW, et al. Fecal microbiota transplant in severe and severe-complicated *Clostridium difficile*: a promising treatment approach. *Gut Microbes.* 2017;8(3):289-302.

4. Ianiro G, Masucci L, Quaranta G, et al. Randomised clinical trial: faecal microbiota transplantation by colonoscopy plus vancomycin for the treatment of severe refractory *Clostridium difficile* infection-single versus multiple infusions. *Aliment Pharmacol Ther.* 2018;48(2):152-159.

5. van Nood E, Vrieze A, Nieuwdorp M, et al. Duodenal infusion of donor feces for recurrent *Clostridium difficile*. *N Engl J Med.* 2013;368(5):407-415.

6. Kelly CR, Khoruts A, Staley C, et al. Effect of fecal microbiota transplantation on recurrence in multiply recurrent *Clostridium difficile* infection: a randomized trial. *Ann Intern Med.* 2016;165(9):609-616.

7. Cammarota G, Masucci L, Ianiro G, et al. Randomised clinical trial: faecal microbiota transplantation by colonoscopy vs. vancomycin for the treatment of recurrent *Clostridium difficile* infection. *Aliment Pharmacol Ther.* 2015;41(9):835-843.

8. Hvas CL, Dahl Jørgensen SM, Jørgensen SP, et al. Fecal microbiota transplantation is superior to fidaxomicin for treatment of recurrent *Clostridium difficile* infection. *Gastroenterology.* 2019;156(5):1324-1332.e3.

9. Lee CH, Steiner T, Petrof EO, et al. Frozen vs fresh fecal microbiota transplantation and clinical resolution of diarrhea in patients with recurrent *Clostridium difficile* infection: a randomized clinical trial. *JAMA.* 2016;315(2):142-149.

10. Jiang ZD, Ajami NJ, Petrosino JF, et al. Randomised clinical trial: faecal microbiota transplantation for recurrent *Clostridum difficile* infection—fresh, or frozen, or lyophilised microbiota from a small pool of healthy donors delivered by colonoscopy. *Aliment Pharmacol Ther.* 2017;45(7):899-908.

11. Kao D, Roach B, Silva M, et al. Effect of oral capsule- vs colonoscopy-delivered fecal microbiota transplantation on recurrent *Clostridium difficile* infection: a randomized clinical trial. *JAMA.* 2017;318(20):1985-1993.

12. Surawicz CM, Brandt LJ, Binion DG, et al. Guidelines for diagnosis, treatment, and prevention of *Clostridium difficile* infections. *Am J Gastroenterol.* 2013;108(4):478-498.

13. Cammarota G, Ianiro G, Tilg H, et al. European consensus conference on faecal microbiota transplantation in clinical practice. *Gut.* 2017;66(4):569-580.

14. McDonald LC, Gerding DN, Johnson S, et al. Clinical practice guidelines for *Clostridium difficile* infection in adults and children: 2017 update by the Infectious Diseases Society of America (IDSA) and Society for Healthcare Epidemiology of America (SHEA). *Clin Infect Dis.* 2018;66(7):987-994.

15. Jackson M, Olefson S, Machan JT, Kelly CR. A high rate of alternative diagnoses in patients referred for presumed *Clostridium difficile* infection. *J Clin Gastroenterol.* 2016;50(9):742-746.

16. Tariq R, Weatherly RM, Kammer PP, Pardi DS, Khanna S. Experience and outcomes at a specialized *Clostridium difficile* clinical practice. *Mayo Clin Proc Innov Qual Outcomes.* 2017;1(1):49-56.

17. Crobach MJT, Vernon JJ, Loo VG, et al. Understanding *Clostridium difficile* colonization. *Clin Microbiol Rev.* 2018;31(2):e00021-17.

18. Wadhwa A, Al Nahhas MF, Dierkhising RA, et al. High risk of post-infectious irritable bowel syndrome in patients with *Clostridium difficile* infection. *Aliment Pharmacol Ther.* 2016;44(6):576-582.

19. Polage CR, Gyorke CE, Kennedy MA, et al. Overdiagnosis of *Clostridium difficile* infection in the molecular test era. *JAMA Intern Med.* 2015;175(11):1792-1801.

20. Barbut F, Gouot C, Lapidus N, et al. Faecal lactoferrin and calprotectin in patients with *Clostridium difficile* infection: a case-control study. *Eur J Clin Microbiol Infect Dis.* 2017;36:2423-2430.

21. Hota SS, Sales V, Tomlinson G, et al. Oral vancomycin followed by fecal transplantation versus tapering oral vancomycin treatment for recurrent *Clostridium difficile* infection: an open-label, randomized controlled trial. *Clin Infect Dis.* 2017;64(3):265-271. doi:10.1093/cid/ciw731

22. Youngster I, Sauk J, Pindar C, et al. Fecal microbiota transplant for relapsing *Clostridium difficile* infection using a frozen inoculum from unrelated donors: a randomized, open-label, controlled pilot study. *Clin Infect Dis.* 2014;58(11):1515-1522.

23. Jiang ZD, Jenq RR, Ajami NJ, et al. Safety and preliminary efficacy of orally administered lyophilized fecal microbiota product compared with frozen product given by enema for recurrent *Clostridium difficile* infection: a randomized clinical trial. *PLoS One.* 2018;13(11):e0205064. doi:10.1371/journal.pone.0205064

24. Furuya-Kanamori L, Marquess J, Yakob L, et al. Asymptomatic *Clostridium difficile* colonization: epidemiology and clinical implications. *BMC Infect Dis.* 2015;15:51

5

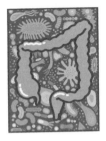

Decision

Considerations for Use of Fecal Microbiota Transplantation in Special Patient Populations

*Rohma Ghani, MBBS, MRCP and
Benjamin H. Mullish, MB, BChir, MRCP, PhD*

As recognition of the utility of fecal microbiota transplantation (FMT) continues to grow, so does the scope of individuals who may potentially benefit from it.[1] Many special patient populations, including pediatric and immunocompromised patients, as well as pregnant patients, were excluded from early FMT clinical trials due to concerns about both the safety and efficacy of using a therapy containing live microorganisms within such patients. However, as experience grows and as longer-term data begin to emerge, there is increasing confidence about the optimal use of FMT in these patient groups. This chapter summarizes unique populations, focusing on the use of FMT for *Clostridioides difficile* infection (CDI; previously *Clostridium difficile*

Allegretti JR, Kassam Z, eds. *The 6 Ds of Fecal
Microbiota Transplantation: A Primer From
Decision to Discharge and Beyond* (pp 43-53).
© 2021 SLACK Incorporated.

infection) and describing the use of FMT for non-CDI indications where experience exists. We will also explore common clinical scenarios that can pose challenges for treating clinicians.

Pediatrics

Diagnosis of CDI in children may present a diagnostic challenge because colonization or transient carriage of *C. difficile*—without true toxin-producing infection—is common, and diarrhea is a common pediatric presentation with multiple possible etiologies. Particular risk factors for CDI in children include antimicrobial and proton-pump inhibitor use, enteral feeding, inflammatory bowel disease (IBD), recent surgery, malignancy, and immunosuppression (eg, due to organ transplantation).[2] Although first-line treatment for pediatric CDI may be broadly similar in approach to adults, there are more notable differences in the treatment of recurrent CDI (rCDI); one relevant issue is that fidaxomicin is not yet approved by the US Food and Drug Administration in children younger than 12 years.[2]

FMT is therefore an attractive alternative option for the treatment of rCDI in children. However, one specific concern regarding the use of FMT in this group has been that the long-term consequences of manipulation of the gut microbiota remain largely unknown. In particular, given the range of clinical conditions in which an association with a perturbed gut microbiota has been described, there is a theoretical concern that the trade-off for successfully treating rCDI in a child with FMT may be transfer of a microbiota trait associated with increased future risk of an alternative condition. However, this remains theoretical, without any evidence that this has occurred in clinical practice.

The largest evidence base to date on FMT in children arises from a recent multicenter retrospective cohort study of 335 patients (age range: 11 months to 23 years) receiving FMT for CDI (Table 5-1).[3] The remission rate after a single FMT was 81%; adverse events were generally similar in frequency and character to those occurring in adult FMT recipients. As such, it has been argued that for children with rCDI, the risk from the known detrimental effects of further antibiotics upon the gut microbiota is typically outweighed by the potential benefits of FMT, despite the currently limited knowledge of any potential long-term impact that FMT may have.[3] In a recent joint position paper from North American and European pediatric gastroenterology societies, the use of FMT following standard-of-care antibiotics was recommended in children with CDI for similar indications to that typically recommended in adults.[2] FMT for children with potential non-CDI indications is a field in which there are a number of ongoing randomized trials, but where experience is generally limited, and no specific recommendations may be made at present.[2]

Table 5-1. Summary of Studies of Fecal Microbiota Transplantation in Special Patient Populations for the Treatment of *Clostridioides difficile* Infection

Use of FMT	No. of Studies	No. of Patients	Pooled Clinical Cure Rate, %[a]	Notes
Pediatrics[3,4]	13	468	85.7	No published randomized trials regarding the use of FMT in children for CDI.
Immunocompromised patients[5]	44	303	87.7	Growing interest in the use of FMT to treat potential sequelae of immunosuppression, including gut graft vs host disease, immune checkpoint inhibitor-related colitis, etc.
Pregnancy[6]	1	1	100	Single case report only.
IBD[7-9]	10	354	80.9	Existing studies are retrospective and heterogeneous in design; the safety and efficacy of FMT in patients with both IBD and CDI is being assessed prospectively in an ongoing study (NCT03106844).

Table includes published studies (excluding abstracts) as of 2020.
[a]Defined variably in different studies, but typically as resolution of CDI-related symptoms at 8 weeks post-FMT.

Immunocompromised Patients

Immunocompromised patients are a group at higher risk of rCDI due to a number of factors, including their impaired humoral immunity and increased need for antibiotics. However, there were initial concerns regarding the safety of using microbiome therapies such as FMT within this vulnerable population. There is now evidence from a small number of patients in a randomized clinical trial,[10] a growing number of case reports and case series,[5,11-14] and a systemic review[15] that collectively demonstrates that, overall, FMT for rCDI is of similar safety and efficacy in patients with a wide variety of immunocompromised states in comparison to immunocompetent individuals (see Table 5-1). The reported literature includes patients with causes of immunocompromise including immunosuppressant agents (eg, chemotherapy, thiopurines, ciclosporin, anti–tumor necrosis factor therapy, corticosteroids), HIV infection (or other inherited or primary immunodeficiency syndromes), end-stage kidney disease, hematologic malignancy or solid organ tumors, or transplant of either a solid organ or bone marrow. Neutropenia does not obviously appear to increase the risk of adverse outcomes from FMT,[12] although experience still remains relatively limited, particularly in the case of severe neutropenia (absolute neutrophil count < 1000/uL). However, this evidence base represents heterogeneous study designs and relatively limited follow-up,[15] and, therefore, the potential suitability of FMT for an immunocompromised recipient should still be considered on a case-by-case basis, balancing potential risk with benefit (Practical Pearl 5-1).

Solid organ transplant (SOT) recipients have been a particular discussion point regarding the suitability for FMT. Previously, when FMT was an emerging practice, the American Society of Transplantation advised against FMT in these patients,[16] outlining theoretical concerns about transferring bacteria into a gut with a disrupted gut mucosal barrier and associated potential risks of bacterial translocation. In 2019, Cheng et al[17] reported on 94 SOT patients who were treated with FMT for CDI. Overall, severe adverse events were noted to be around 3.4%, a rate comparable to the immunocompetent population. However, importantly, it was noted that 3 cytomegalovirus (CMV) seropositive patients underwent CMV reactivation shortly after FMT. These cases are notably different from the previously discussed concern regarding seroconversion in recipients who are negative for CMV. Furthermore, there have been 2 cases of extended-spectrum beta-lactamase (ESBL)–producing *Escherichia coli* bacteremia in immunocompromised recipients (1 patient with cirrhosis and hepatic encephalopathy and 1 following bone marrow transplantation who died) after transmission

Practical Pearl 5-1

When Not to Do a Fecal Microbiota Transplantation

There are clinical situations in which an FMT should typically be avoided, including the following:

- Severe neutropenia (absolute neutrophil count < 1000/uL)
  - Recommend waiting until the patient has neutrophil count recovery
- Perforation or microperforation
- Pregnancy
  - Recommend waiting until after delivery if possible

There are clinical situations in which FMT is not absolutely contraindicated but should be considered thoughtfully, including the following:

- Patients on or frequently receiving systemic antibiotics
  - Counsel the patient on the risk of FMT failure and the likelihood of requiring more than 1 FMT
- Older patients with limited life expectancy
- Allergist-confirmed food-related anaphylaxis
  - Recommend using a patient-directed donor with food eliminated from diet

from an ESBL *E. coli*–colonized donor.[18,19] Importantly, the donor had not undergone appropriate ESBL stool testing, emphasizing the importance of screening for intestinal colonization of multi-drug–resistant organisms in all potential donors (see Chapter 6: "Donor: How Do You Select and Screen Candidate Donors for Fecal Microbiota Transplantation?").[20-23]

Immunocompromised patients should be considered candidates for FMT for recurrent, refractory, severe, and fulminant CDI. In patients who are severely immunocompromised (eg, organ transplant recipients on multiple immunosuppressive agents) and test negative for CMV, a CMV-negative donor should be identified if possible, and the patient should be counseled that risks of infection may be higher if the donor is CMV positive. It may be clinically rational to defer FMT until after completion of chemotherapy in cancer patients with multiply rCDI who remain asymptomatic during treatment with vancomycin.

Clostridioides difficile Infection and Inflammatory Bowel Disease

Rates of CDI in patients with IBD, particularly those with ulcerative colitis, may be up to 8-fold higher than in patients without IBD.[24] Furthermore, patients with IBD who develop CDI are more likely to develop adverse health outcomes, including higher rates of IBD flares, longer hospital stays, more CDI recurrences, and increased rates of failure of medical therapy for IBD, need for surgery, and mortality.[24] Treatment of CDI in patients with IBD itself presents particular challenges, including difficulty in distinguishing an IBD flare from CDI and uncertainty about the appropriateness of continuation of potent immunosuppressive IBD therapy during treatment for CDI.[24] Confirming active CDI in IBD patients is often a challenge that complicates the decision to perform FMT, particularly because it is not always clear whether symptoms are related to the *C. difficile* or the underlying disease process. Because a *C. difficile* polymerase chain reaction (PCR) assay does not distinguish colonization from active infection, one may consider using the more specific toxin enzyme immunoassay; however, some clinicians feel the presence of *C. difficile* in the setting of disease flare is an indication for standard-of-care CDI antibiotics, whether or not the toxin is detectable. CDI may exacerbate IBD activity, which often adds to the dilemma of decision and timing of FMT; therefore, we recommend optimization of IBD medications to eliminate that as a potential confounder. In addition, given the higher likelihood of adverse outcomes with CDI in IBD patients, FMT may be considered after 2 or more CDI episodes, even without history of severe CDI disease.

The initial data regarding outcomes of FMT in the treatment of CDI in patients with IBD were retrospective in nature. These data demonstrated overall reduced efficacy at preventing CDI recurrence in patients with IBD, with reports of IBD flare rates between 18% and 54%, although flares were poorly defined.[25-27] In contrast, a subsequent systematic review of randomized clinical trials and high-quality studies in which FMT had been administered to patients with IBD identified much lower rates of worsening of IBD activity, reported as 4.6% (see Table 5-1).[7,28] One potential explanation for the apparent disparity between these results from retrospective and randomized studies may have been the use of *C. difficile* PCR testing in the former group and potential misattribution of IBD flares as CDI episodes. A prospective multicenter cohort study of FMT in patients with rCDI and comorbid IBD by Allegretti et al[29] reported high rates of clinical cure of

CDI, in keeping with cure rates in non-IBD patients, and also noted IBD disease activity improvement. There was only a single case of an IBD de novo flare (1/50) reported. Overall, FMT is felt to be safe and effective for the treatment of CDI in patients with IBD, but patients should be counseled about a small potential risk of disease flare.[20] In IBD, a lower gastrointestinal route of administration is preferred because it may help assess IBD disease activity at the time of FMT. IBD patients with CDI may not have classic pseudomembranes, even in severe cases. Nonresponsive patients should also be assessed for alternate etiologies, including opportunistic infections, concomitant celiac disease, common variable immunodeficiency, or other immunodeficiency states. Routine mucosal biopsies should also be obtained to assess histologic disease activity at time of FMT, particularly in patients with inflammation on endoscopy to rule out CMV infection, and especially in patients on biologic agents or other immunosuppressive therapy. The existing evidence supports referral for FMT in IBD patients with rCDI and is supported by experts in best practice guidelines.[22]

Pregnancy

There is limited experience regarding the use of FMT in this patient population. One case report describes successful administration of FMT for CDI in a pregnant patient at 18 weeks' gestation via colonoscopy. Her symptoms resolved after a single FMT, with normal delivery of the baby at 39 weeks.[6] Most authorities would recommend avoiding FMT during pregnancy unless there was a very compelling indication for its consideration.

Food Allergy and Anaphylaxis

Concerns have been raised regarding the potential triggering of food allergies in patients who receive stool from donors who may have food allergens for that recipient in their diet, and therefore also potentially within their stool. To date, there does not appear to be any published reports of an anaphylactic reaction post-FMT; however, most FMT studies have excluded potential recipients with a history of severe food allergy/anaphylaxis, and this is still viewed as at least a relative contraindication to receiving FMT from a universal donor in some clinical guidelines.[20,30]

Where there is uncertainty as to whether a potential FMT recipient has a true food allergy, one approach may be referral for evaluation by an allergist for confirmation.[28] Should the allergy be confirmed, clinicians could consider preparing the FMT from the stool of a patient-identified donor who has omitted the potential allergens from their diet for 1 week.[28] Similarly, where a recipient has celiac disease, it may be reasonable to consider FMT preparation from a patient-identified donor on a gluten-free diet.[20]

Conversely, there is growing interest in the potential contribution of gut microbiota–host immune system interactions to the development of food allergy, and a Phase 1 open-label trial is in place to evaluate the use of FMT by capsule in the treatment of peanut allergy.[31]

Concomitant Antibiotics

One challenging scenario for clinicians is the administration of FMT to patients with rCDI who also have a strong indication for long-term, non-CDI antibiotics (eg, splenectomy, osteomyelitis), or recipients who develop a non-CDI–related indication that requires antibiotics shortly after receiving FMT. In this scenario, the central concern is that the use of antimicrobials may reduce engraftment of FMT-derived microbial communities within the host and, therefore, limit its effectiveness. Furthermore, there is now supporting evidence that this may also be the case in clinical practice; for instance, approximately 50% of the FMT failures from the Dutch Donor Feces Bank in preventing rCDI occurred in patients receiving antibiotics within 1 month of their FMT.[30] In addition, a retrospective study demonstrated that use of non–anti-CDI antibiotics within 8 weeks of FMT is associated with an approximately 3-fold risk of FMT failure.[32]

One clinical message from such studies is to only administer non-CDI antibiotics to FMT recipients within the early post-FMT period (ie, up to 8 weeks) when there is a compelling indication. Where non-CDI antibiotics cannot be avoided, liaison with infectious disease/medical microbiology specialists is recommended to attempt to identify the most "microbiota-protective" antimicrobial regimen possible.[20]

Summary

As the evidence base continues to grow, the potential utility of FMT also increases. To date, studies evaluating FMT in special populations have predominantly consisted of heterogeneous retrospective case series, and gaps in knowledge are therefore still wide. Reassuringly, efficacy of FMT for CDI in these populations appears generally similar to conventional recipients, and the reported rates of serious adverse events still appear to be low overall. Hopefully this will translate to such patients being included in future FMT trials where they may previously have been ineligible. The establishment of national FMT registries, such as those established in the United States[33] and Germany,[34] will also provide a valuable resource for the further evaluation of the long-term safety and efficacy of FMT in special populations.

References

1. Allegretti JR, Mullish BH, Kelly C, Fischer M. The evolution of the use of faecal microbiota transplantation and emerging therapeutic indications. *Lancet.* 2019;394(10196):420-431.

2. Davidovics ZH, Michail S, Nicholson MR, et al. Fecal microbiota transplantation for recurrent *Clostridium difficile* infection and other conditions in children: a joint position paper from the North American Society for Pediatric Gastroenterology, Hepatology, and Nutrition and the European Society for Pediatric Gastroenterology, Hepatology, and Nutrition. *J Pediatr Gastroenterol Nutr.* 2019;68(1):130-143.

3. Nicholson MR, Mitchell PD, Alexander E, et al. Efficacy of fecal microbiota transplantation for *Clostridium difficile* infection in children. *Clin Gastroenterol Hepatol.* 2020;18(3):612-619.e1.

4. Hourigan SK, Oliva-Hemker M. Fecal microbiota transplantation in children: a brief review. *Pediatr Res.* 2016;80(1):2-6.

5. Abu-Sbeih H, Ali FS, Wang Y. Clinical review on the utility of fecal microbiota transplantation in immunocompromised patients. *Curr Gastroenterol Rep.* 2019;21(3):8.

6. Saeedi BJ, Morison DG, Kraft CS, Dhere T. Fecal microbiota transplant for *Clostridium difficile* infection in a pregnant patient. *Obstet Gynecol.* 2017;129(3):507-509.

7. Qazi T, Amaratunga T, Barnes EL, Fischer M, Kassam Z, Allegretti JR. The risk of inflammatory bowel disease flares after fecal microbiota transplantation: systematic review and meta-analysis. *Gut Microbes.* 2017;8(6):574-588.

8. Chen T, Zhou Q, Zhang D, et al. Effect of faecal microbiota transplantation for treatment of *Clostridium difficile* infection in patients with inflammatory bowel disease: a systematic review and meta-analysis of cohort studies. *J Crohn's Colitis.* 2018;12(6):710-717

9. Cho S, Spencer E, Hirten R, Grinspan A, Dubinsky MC. Fecal microbiota transplant for recurrent *Clostridium difficile* infection in pediatric inflammatory bowel disease. *J Pediatr Gastroenterol Nutr.* 2019;68(3):343-347.

10. Lee CH, Steiner T, Petrof EO, et al. Frozen vs fresh fecal microbiota transplantation and clinical resolution of diarrhea in patients with recurrent *Clostridium difficile* infection a randomized clinical trial. *JAMA.* 2016;315(2):142-149.

11. Rubin TA, Gessert CE, Aas J, Bakken JS. Fecal microbiome transplantation for recurrent *Clostridium difficile* infection: report on a case series. *Anaerobe.* 2013;19:22-26.

12. Hefazi M, Patnaik MM, Hogan WJ, Litzow MR, Pardi DS, Khanna S. Safety and efficacy of fecal microbiota transplant for recurrent *Clostridium difficile* infection in patients with cancer treated with cytotoxic chemotherapy: a single-institution retrospective case series. *Mayo Clin Proc.* 2017;92(11):1617-1624.

13. Agrawal M, Aroniadis OC, Brandt LJ, et al. The long-term efficacy and safety of fecal microbiota transplant for recurrent, severe, and complicated *Clostridium difficile* infection in 146 elderly individuals. *J Clin Gastroenterol.* 2015;50(5):403-407.

14. Kelly CR, Ihunnah C, Fischer M, et al. Fecal microbiota transplant for treatment of *Clostridium difficile* infection in immunocompromised patients. *Am J Gastroenterol.* 2014;109(7):1065-1071.

15. Shogbesan O, Poudel DR, Victor S, et al. A systematic review of the efficacy and safety of fecal microbiota transplant for *Clostridium difficile* infection in immunocompromised patients. *Can J Gastroenterol Hepatol.* 2018;2018:1-10.

16. Dubberke ER, Burdette SD; AST Infectious Diseases Community of Practice. *Clostridium difficile* infections in solid organ transplantation. *Am J Transplant.* 2013;13(suppl 4):42-49.

17. Cheng YW, Phelps E, Ganapini V, et al. Fecal microbiota transplantation for the treatment of recurrent and severe *Clostridium difficile* infection in solid organ transplant recipients: a multicenter experience. *Am J Transplant.* 2019;19(2):501-511.

18. US Food and Drug Administration. Important safety alert regarding use of fecal microbiota for transplantation and risk of serious adverse reactions due to transmission of multi-drug resistant organisms. June 13, 2019. Accessed June 13, 2020. https://www.fda.gov/vaccines-blood-biologics/safety-availability-biologics/important-safety-alert-regarding-use-fecal-microbiota-transplantation-and-risk-serious-adverse

19. US Food and Drug Administration. Fecal microbiota for transplantation: safety communication – risk of serious adverse reactions due to transmission of multidrug resistant organisms. June 13, 2019. Updated June 18, 2019. Accessed June 13, 2020. https://www.fda.gov/safety/medwatch-safety-alerts-human-medical-products/fecal-microbiota-transplantation-safety-communication-risk-serious-adverse-reactions-due

20. Mullish BH, Quraishi MN, Segal JP, et al. The use of faecal microbiota transplant as treatment for recurrent or refractory *Clostridium difficile* infection and other potential indications: joint British Society of Gastroenterology (BSG) and Healthcare Infection Society (HIS) guidelines. *Gut.* 2018;67(11):1920-1941.

21. Cammarota G, Ianiro G, Tilg H, et al. European consensus conference on faecal microbiota transplantation in clinical practice. *Gut.* 2017;66(4):569-580.

22. Kassam Z, Dubois N, Ramakrishna B, et al. Donor screening for fecal microbiota transplantation. *N Engl J Med.* 2019;381(21):2070-2072.

23. DeFilipp Z, Bloom PP, Torres Soto M, et al. Drug-resistant *E. coli* bacteremia transmitted by fecal microbiota transplant. *N Engl J Med.* 2019;381(21):2043-2050.

24. Khanna S, Shin A, Kelly CP. Management of *Clostridium difficile* infection in inflammatory bowel disease: expert review from the Clinical Practice Updates Committee of the AGA Institute. *Clin Gastroenterol Hepatol.* 2017;15(2):166-174.

25. Khoruts A, Rank KM, Newman KM, et al. Inflammatory bowel disease affects the outcome of fecal microbiota transplantation for recurrent *Clostridium difficile* infection. *Clin Gastroenterol Hepatol.* 2016;14(10):1433-1438.

26. Chin SM, Sauk J, Mahabamunuge J, Kaplan JL, Hohmann EL, Khalili H. Fecal microbiota transplantation for recurrent *Clostridium difficile* infection in patients with inflammatory bowel disease: a single-center experience. *Clin Gastroenterol Hepatol.* 2017;15(4):597-599.

27. Fischer M, Kao D, Kelly C, et al. Fecal microbiota transplantation is safe and efficacious for recurrent or refractory *Clostridium difficile* infection in patients with inflammatory bowel disease. *Inflamm Bowel Dis.* 2016;22(10):2402-2409.

28. Allegretti JR, Kassam Z, Osman M, Budree S, Fischer M, Kelly CR. The 5D framework: a clinical primer for fecal microbiota transplantation to treat *Clostridium difficile* infection. *Gastrointest Endosc.* 2018;87(1):18-29.

29. Allegretti JR, Kelly CR, Grinspan A, et al. Outcomes of fecal microbiota transplantation in patients with inflammatory bowel diseases and recurrent *Clostridioides difficile* infection. *Gastroenterology.* 2020;s0016-5085(20)35008-3.

30. Terveer EM, van Beurden YH, Goorhuis A, et al. How to: establish and run a stool bank. *Clin Microbiol Infect.* 2017;23(12):924-930.

31. Zhao W, Ho HE, Bunyavanich S. The gut microbiome in food allergy. *Ann Allergy Asthma Immunol.* 2019;122(3):276-282.

32. Allegretti JR, Kao D, Sitko J, Fischer M, Kassam Z. Early antibiotic use post-fecal microbiota transplantation increases the risk of treatment failure. *Clin Infect Dis.* 2017;66(1):134-135.

33. Kelly CR, Kim AM, Laine L, Wu GD. The AGA's Fecal Microbiota Transplantation National Registry: an important step toward understanding risks and benefits of microbiota therapeutics. *Gastroenterology.* 2017;152(4):681-684.

34. Peri R, Aguilar RC, Tüffers K, et al. The impact of technical and clinical factors on fecal microbiota transfer outcomes for the treatment of recurrent *Clostridioides difficile* infections in Germany. *United European Gastroenterol J.* 2019;7(5):716-722.

6

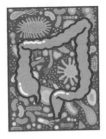

Donor

How Do You Select and Screen Candidate Donors for Fecal Microbiota Transplantation?

Shrish Budree, MBChB, DCH, FCPaeds, Cert. Paeds Gastro.

The selection and screening of a donor is one of the most important steps to ensure that fecal microbiota transplantation (FMT) is as safe as possible. Broadly, there are 2 general approaches to identifying an appropriate donor: patient-selected and universal. Donor screening is one of the more challenging aspects of the FMT process, both clinically and logistically.[1] In this chapter we will review the best available evidence with regard to how to select stool donors as well as appropriate screening procedures.

Allegretti JR, Kassam Z, eds. *The 6 Ds of Fecal Microbiota Transplantation: A Primer From Decision to Discharge and Beyond* (pp 55-70).
© 2021 SLACK Incorporated.

Patient-Selected Donors

In the patient-selected donor model, the donor is known to the patient and may be a close relative, spouse, or friend. The candidate donor is identified by the patient, and the treating physician will be required to screen the donor and collect and process their material before performing the FMT procedure. Should the candidate donor not pass the screening tests, another donor will need to be sought, which may be time-consuming. Historically, this model was the most common approach for FMT donor section, and it is still used by some centers today.[2,3]

The advantages of patient-selected donors include a higher likelihood of the donor sharing a similar microbiome profile as the recipient; reduced risk of exposure to allergy-triggering antigens in the stool of donors who are from the same household, often perceived as more acceptable by patients when they know the person who donated the material; and less risk of a donor-related adverse event affecting multiple recipients (Practical Pearl 6-1).[4] However, there are a number of limitations with the patient-selected model, including ethical concerns about coercion and lack of voluntary admission of engagement in risky behavior associated with infectious diseases; the high costs associated with screening donors, which may not be covered by the patient's medical insurance and may lead to physicians performing fewer screening tests; more physician-related barriers, such as the processing of donor material; and the delay in obtaining material for treatment.[1]

Universal Donors

Following expansion of knowledge in the FMT field showing similar efficacy for fresh vs frozen material in recurrent *Clostridioides difficile* infection (CDI) and the growth of the stool bank model, most centers in the United States and Europe now use universal stool donor material to treat their patients. In the universal donor model, the stool donor is not known to the patient, similar to a blood bank. Donors are sourced and thoroughly screened by the stool bank (Figure 6-1). Once donors have successfully passed the screening process, they donate material regularly and the material is processed and stored in -80° C freezers until requested by the physician. Upon request, the material can be shipped under temperature control to the treating center (Practical Pearl 6-2).

The advantages of the universal stool donor model include more rapid access to material to treat the patient, particularly for severe and fulminant CDI; thoroughly screened donors; lower overall system costs;

Practical Pearl 6-1

Are There Scenarios Where Patient-Selected Stool Donation Would Be Preferred?

There are several scenarios where you and the patient may feel more comfortable using a patient-directed stool donor as opposed to a universal donor. These include the following:

- Severe food-related allergy/anaphylaxis: If the patient has anaphylactoid allergies to any food substance, first confirm this allergy with an allergist if there is any clinical uncertainty. If medically confirmed, consider using a patient-selected donor and advise the donor to avoid that allergen. General guidance is avoidance for at least 1 week; however, there are no data to guide the ideal time.
- Cytomegalovirus (CMV)– and Epstein-Barr virus (EBV)–negative immunocompromised: If a patient is immunocompromised and has never been exposed to CMV or EBV (ie, serum immunoglobulin G [IgG] levels are negative for CMV or EBV), you may want to consider using a donor that has also never been exposed to CMV or EBV. Epidemiology data suggest the majority of donors have a history of EBV and CMV exposure; therefore, it is not part of routine donor screening, and there would be a theoretical risk of CMV- or EBV-associated infection in a vulnerable patient.
- Pregnancy: FMT in a pregnancy should be avoided if possible; however, if strongly indicated, using the pregnant patient's partner as the donor is the recommended approach.

centralized quality control and safety monitoring of the FMT material; and fewer barriers for physicians and patients to access safe material for treatment. One limitation with this model includes the risk of affecting multiple recipients if there is a donor-related adverse event (eg, the donor is found to be colonized by a pathogenic organism).

Donor Consent

Stool donation must be voluntary. Donors should be informed about the risks and benefits of becoming a stool donor and provide written informed consent. Prior to signing the consent form, donors should be made aware of the detailed screening process and the possibility of incidental findings, and measures should be taken to ensure donor confidentiality. Candidate donors will need to be consented for screening and commit to providing truthful answers to medical

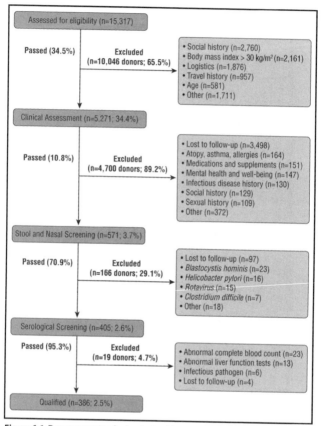

Figure 6-1. Donor screening for fecal microbiota transplantation and qualification rate of candidate donors. (Adapted from Kassam et al.[5])

Practical Pearl 6-2

What Are the Differences Between the Universal Donor and the Patient-Selected Models?

Universal

Safety
- Standardized, comprehensive screening.
- Accounts for seroconversion delay.
- Centralized adverse events reporting and auditing.
- Possible risk of donor transmitting disease to many patients.

Access
- No physician time or expertise required to locate and screen qualified donors.
- No time or expertise needed for material preparation.
- For all universal donation, no delay in patient care.
- Enables broad patient access.

Cost
- Lower overall cost to the system.
- Predictable costs to obtain donor material.

Patient-Selected

Safety
- Screening variability between providers.
- Potentially less comprehensive screening.
- Voluntary adverse events reporting.
- Risk of donor transmitting disease is contained to a small patient population.

Access
- Physician needs time and expertise to locate and screen qualified donors.
- Time and expertise needed for material preparation.
- Potential delay in patient care.
- Likely limited to academic centers where comprehensive screening can be performed.

Cost
- Higher overall cost to the system (1 donor per patient).
- Unpredictable costs to obtain donor material.

*Universal donor associated with stool bank.

Adapted from Edelstein et al.[6]

questionnaires. In addition, the consent should include specific sections on material storage for future safety testing and sequencing analysis.

Donor Screening

Medical History Screening

Candidate donors should undergo detailed medical history, infectious disease risk assessment, and clinical evaluation for possible microbiome-mediated diseases. It should be noted that, similar to blood banking, there is limited direct evidence on the need to screen for these specific types of conditions; however, the recommendations that follow are current best practice based on expert opinion and guideline statements. Donors should be healthy without gastrointestinal (GI) disease and on no antibiotics in the 3 months prior to donation.[7,8] Clinical questionnaires are usually based on blood bank or organ transplant questionnaires and are aimed at assessing infectious disease risk in candidate donors. Questions should focus on travel history to countries with endemic diseases, use of illicit drugs, and high-risk sexual behavior. In addition, the clinical assessment should be directed at determining the presence of known microbiome-mediated disease. There are currently several diseases that have been associated with the microbiome. Although the directionality of causation remains to be fully understood, there are data to suggest associations with autoimmune disease, atopy, inflammatory bowel disease (IBD), colorectal cancer, chronic pain syndromes (eg, fibromyalgia, chronic fatigue), neurologic or neurodevelopmental disorders, certain neuropsychiatric conditions, metabolic syndrome, and obesity.[9,10] Personal history of such diseases should exclude candidate donors. The donor clinical assessment should include weight, height, abdominal circumference, body mass index (BMI), and general systems assessment. Donor age is an important consideration with most centers, with ages ranging from 18 to 50 years, because the microbiome is most stable during this time of life.[11,12] A framework for a candidate clinical questionnaire is provided in Table 6-1.

Stool and Serological Testing

Candidate donors who pass the initial clinical assessment screen should undergo serological and stool testing, predominantly aimed at excluding transmissible infectious diseases (Table 6-2).

Baseline Metabolic Tests

Some centers recommend performing baseline hematology, electrolyte, renal function, liver function, and inflammatory marker tests on donors (see Table 6-2). Clinically significant abnormalities in these baseline tests may excluded candidate donors depending on the underlying etiology of the test abnormality. The significance of raised nonspecific inflammatory markers such as C-reactive protein and fecal calprotectin in an asymptomatic healthy individual is unknown, so the utility of this test remains questionable.

Infectious Disease Panel

Recommendations for testing vary slightly from one guideline to another based on local disease prevalence; however, there are certain mandatory tests that must be performed in all donors that are consistent across guidelines. These include testing for HIV, hepatitis A, hepatitis B, hepatitis C, syphilis, and *Strongyloides*. Mandatory stool testing includes screening for antibiotic-resistant bacteria (ARB; vancomycin-resistant *Enterococcus* [VRE], extended-spectrum beta-lactamase [ESBL]–producing organisms, carbapenem-resistant *Enterobacteriaceae* [CRE], and methicillin-resistant *Staphylococcus aureus* [MRSA; nasal swab permissible]), common enteric pathogens, *C. difficile*, *Giardia lamblia*, *Cryptosporidium*, *Isospora*, and *Microsporidia* and examination for ova and parasites.[3,9-11] Tests that vary across guidelines include testing donor stool for viruses (adenovirus, norovirus, rotavirus). *Helicobacter pylori* fecal antigen has been recommended for upper route delivery.[8]

In June 2019, the US Food and Drug Administration (FDA) released a safety alert after an FMT-related death of an immunocompromised patient from ESBL bacteremia from a hospital FMT program that did not appropriately screen donors.[13] The FDA guidance following this unfortunate event advises that all donors be screened for increased risk of ARB colonization such as health care workers, extended hospital admissions, persons residing in long-term care facilities, persons who frequently attend outpatient units, and those who engage in medical tourism. In addition, all donor stool must be tested for ARBs such as VRE, ESBL, CRE, and MRSA (nasal/peri-rectal swab permissible).

Recommendations for testing for CMV and EBV in donors vary. A large proportion of the healthy adults are exposed to these viruses with positive serology (IgG), and this could lead to the inappropriate exclusion of healthy donors.[9,10] To date, there are no documented cases of CMV/EBV transmission related to FMT. Therefore, donors should not be excluded if they are CMV/EBV exposed (ie, IgG positive). Special consideration should be given to immunocompromised populations at risk of CMV/EBV disease who are receiving an FMT. These recipients should be tested to determine whether they are

Table 6-1. Clinical Assessment for Donor Screening

	Clinical Screening Criteria
Medical History of, or Risk Factors for, Infectious Diseases	• History of HIV, hepatitis B or C viruses, syphilis, human T-lymphotropic virus I and II • Current systemic infection • Use of illegal drugs • High-risk sexual behavior • Previous tissue/organ transplant • Recent hospitalization or discharge from long-term care facilities • High-risk travel/engaged in medical tourism • Recent (≤6 months) needle stick accident • Recent (≤6 months) body tattoo, piercing, acupuncture • Recent (≤2 months) enteric pathogen infection • Recent (≤2 months) acute gastroenteritis with or without confirmatory test • History of receiving growth hormone, insulin from cows, or clotting factor concentrates • Recent (≤2 months) history of vaccination with a live attenuated virus, if there is a possible risk of transmission **Demographics That Impact the Microbiome** • Age 18 to 50 years **Employment** • Health care worker with patient exposure or other risk factors for colonization by multi-drug resistant organisms

(continued)

Table 6-1 (continued). Clinical Assessment for Donor Screening

	Clinical Screening Criteria
Disorders Potentially Associated With Perturbation of the Gut Microbiota	• Personal history of chronic GI disease, including functional GI disorders, IBD, celiac disease, other chronic gastroenterological diseases • Personal history of systemic autoimmune disorders • Personal history of cancer, including GI cancers or polyposis syndrome • Recent abnormal GI symptoms (eg, diarrhea, hematochezia) • Personal history of neurological/neurodegenerative disorders • Personal history of psychiatric/neurodevelopmental conditions • Obesity (BMI > 30 kg/m^2) and/or metabolic syndrome/diabetes • First-degree family history of premature colon cancer or first-degree family history of early-onset polyposis syndrome
Drugs That Can Alter Gut Microbiota	• Recent (≤3 months) exposure to systemic antimicrobial drugs, immunosuppressant agents, chemotherapy • Chronic treatment (≥3 months) with daily use of proton pump inhibitors

Adapted from Cammarota et al.[10]

Table 6-2. Donor Testing: International Expert Consensus Guidelines and FDA Considerations for Screening

	Rome Guidelines[10]	FDA Considerations[14,a]
Blood	- Hepatitis A, hepatitis B, hepatitis C, and hepatitis E viruses - HIV-1/2 - Treponema pallidum - Nematodes (Strongyloides stercoralis) - Complete blood cell count with differential - Creatinine - Aminotransferases, bilirubin	- Hepatitis A, hepatitis B, hepatitis C - HIV-1/2 - Human T-lymphotropic virus 1/2 - T. pallidum - Strongyloides - CMV (depending on patient population)
Stool	- C. difficile - Common enteric pathogens, including Salmonella, Shigella, Campylobacter, Shiga toxin–producing E. coli (STEC), Yersinia, and Vibrio cholerae - ARB, including VRE and MRSA; gram-negative ARB, including ESBL-producing Enterobacteriaceae and carbapenemase-producing Enterobacteriaceae (CRE)	- C. difficile - Salmonella spp, Shigella spp, Campylobacter spp, E. coli 0157, Yersinia spp, and Vibrio spp - Plesiomonas spp - Multi-drug-resistant organisms, including VRE, ESBL-producing Enterobacteriaceae, CRE, MRSA (nasal/peri-rectal swab permissible) - Norovirus, rotavirus, adenovirus, enterovirus - Giardia - Cryptosporidium, Cyclospora, Isospora, Microsporidia (continued)

Table 6-2 (continued). Donor Testing: International Expert Consensus Guidelines and FDA Considerations for Screening

	Rome Guidelines[10]	FDA Considerations[14,a]
Stool	• Norovirus, rotavirus, adenovirus • *Giardia lamblia, Cryptosporidium* spp, *Isospora, Microsporidia* • Protozoa and helminths/ova and parasites (including *Blastocystis hominis* and *Dientamoeba fragilis*) • *H. pylori* fecal antigen (for upper route of FMT delivery)	• *Entamoeba histolytica* • Ova and parasites
Emerging	• Severe acute respiratory syndrome coronavirus 2 (SARS-CoV-2)	• SARS-CoV-2

[a]The FDA notes that donor testing protocols may differ from this list for a number of reasons, including, but not limited to, indication and clinical context of recipient population (eg, severely immunocompromised).

Adapted from Cammarota et al[10] and Caralson.[14]

seronegative, and, if so, a seronegative donor should be sought or the recipient should be thoroughly counseled about the risk of CMV/EBV-associated transmission through FMT.

In March 2020, the FDA issued a safety alert following the possible transmission of STEC to 4 patients and enteropathogenic E. coli (EPEC) to 2 severely immunocompromised patients who received FMT. The outcome was transient diarrhea, and all 6 patients' symptoms resolved. These were the first reported cases of infection associated with these organisms following FMT. Based on this information, the FDA now requires that all donor material is tested for STEC using validated molecular testing techniques (polymerase chain reaction [PCR] testing). Although testing for the highly virulent STEC has been part of existing FMT guidelines, the type of test has not been specified, and toxin enzyme immunoassay testing has been determined to not be sufficiently sensitive. Accordingly, we recommend STEC testing by PCR for donor screening programs.

The FDA's recommendation to conduct EPEC testing by molecular testing is controversial. No guidelines recommend testing for EPEC. In addition, EPEC testing may not be applicable in all countries or patient populations. This is due to the lack of information regarding the virulence potential of this organism and data suggesting it is commonly found as part of the normal gut commensal community in healthy individuals.[7] Further characterization of specific virulent EPEC strains and development of validated methods for testing for these strains is required. Exclusion of susceptible individuals at risk for EPEC infection, such as severely immunocompromised patients (eg, primary Ig deficiencies) may also be a consideration.[7]

Emerging Pathogen

Coronavirus disease 2019 (COVID-19) is caused by a novel coronavirus, SARS-CoV-2, and was designated a pandemic by the World Health Organization in March 2020.[8] The clinical manifestations of this condition range from asymptomatic infection to severe pneumonia with respiratory failure, and it is associated with a high mortality rate in older individuals. Several recent studies have documented the presence of SARS-CoV-2 RNA and/or SARS-CoV-2 virus in stool of infected individuals, suggesting that SARS-CoV-2 may be transmitted by FMT.[15]

Based on this information, the FDA released a Medwatch Safety Alert in March 2020, recommending the following additional testing of donors and donor stool produced after December 1, 2019. First, they suggested that additional clinical screening of donors include questions directed at identifying those who may be currently or recently infected with SARS-CoV-2. Second, they suggested testing donors and/or donor stool for SARS-CoV-2. At present, there are no validated tests for detecting virus in stool; therefore, donor screening programs are currently testing donors using validated nasal pharyngeal swab testing. This recommendation is consistent with an international expert panel that commented on donor screening during the COVID-19 outbreak.[16]

Continuous Assessment of Universal Donors

Universal donors who are part of a stool bank should have ongoing health screens and infectious disease testing performed to ensure their material remains safe for use in FMT. There are various strategies employed by stool banks and guideline recommendations for continuous health monitoring. A large US stool bank performs brief health assessments at each donation, repeats stool and serological testing every 6 weeks, and quarantines material produced (to address seroconversion windows) during these 6-week blocks until the donor test results before and after the 6-week block are determine to be normal.[3,9] An international consensus guideline similarly recommends the administration of a clinical questionnaire on the day of donation and the performance of repeat clinical assessment and laboratory testing every 8 to 12 weeks.[10] The ideal frequency of stool testing is unknown, and for maximum safety each individual stool should be tested, as opposed to only testing before a donating block. After the donating block is complete, release of the quarantined material is required.

Additional Considerations Regarding Fecal Microbiota Transplantation Donor Screening

Laboratory Testing

Validated laboratory testing should be performed and should be guided by local and regional guidelines. It may be important to discuss testing options with local labs to avoid samples being rejected, specifically with regard to GI infectious disease testing of formed stool.

Pediatric Populations and Age-Matched Donors

Currently, most guidelines recommend adult donors because there has not been a concerning safety profile using adult donors for pediatric patients. A large multicenter pediatric study (N = 335) reported an 81% clinical cure rate after a single FMT predominantly using adult stool donors with a tolerable safety profile.[17] However, children and adolescents exhibit a distinct microbial profile compared with adults.[12] Accordingly, the transfer of an adult microbiome into a child could potentially impact efficacy of the transplantation (a child's intestinal tract is both anatomically and physiologically different from an adult's) and normal maturation of the child's microbiome, leading to potential future effects on the child's health. Therefore, some experts in the field have recommended further research into age-matched donors, specifically related to FMT within the pediatric population.

Fecal Microbiota Transplantation in Patients With Significant Allergy

Special consideration should be given to careful selection of donors for patients with a history of anaphylaxis or anaphylactoid reactions. There is the possibility that stool could contain antigens that trigger an allergic reaction; however, no related cases have been described to date. Patient-selected donors may be a better option in these complex cases.

The Future of Donor Screening in Fecal Microbiota Transplantation

The concept of a *super-donor* has emerged in the context of FMT studies in ulcerative colitis. In 2 separate randomized clinical trials, 1 out of approximately 5 to 10 donors was found to be associated with higher rates of disease remission compared with the other donors.[18,19] This raised the possibility of a *donor effect*, which hypothesizes that certain donors have a superior or healthier microbial community that is more effective in a specific disease. Large observation cohort data from a US stool bank suggest there is no donor effect in CDI; however, more research is required to explore diseases where there may be super-donors. Overall, this is an intriguing question and could lead to a future where donors are selected not only based on their safety profile but also their microbial community composition.

Summary

In-depth donor screening is imperative to safety in FMT, irrespective of whether material is sourced from a patient-selected or a universal donor. Although current guidelines are based on limited evidence and are predominantly expert driven, they exist to help direct physicians through the donor selection process. There are core consensus clinical screening and laboratory tests that should be performed in all candidate donors. Data continue to emerge on the screening process, and there remains some variability in practice, so

FMT clinicians should be mindful of this evolving area. Overall, similar to blood banking, this field will likely continue to change as we move toward evidence-based consensus screening guidelines.

References

1. Bakken JS, Polgreen PM, Beekmann SE, Riedo FX, Streit JA. Treatment approaches including fecal microbiota transplantation for recurrent *Clostridium difficile* infection (RCDI) among infectious disease physicians. *Anaerobe.* 2013;24:20-24.

2. Lee CH, Steiner T, Petrof EO, et al. Frozen vs fresh fecal microbiota transplantation and clinical resolution of diarrhea in patients with recurrent *Clostridium difficile* infection: a randomized clinical trial. *JAMA.* 2016;315(2):142-149.

3. Panchal P, Budree S, Scheeler A, et al. Scaling safe access to fecal microbiota transplantation: past, present, and future. *Curr Gastroenterol Rep.* 2018;20(4):14.

4. Dill-McFarland KA, Tang ZZ, Kemis JH, et al. Close social relationships correlate with human gut microbiota composition. *Sci Rep.* 2019;9:703.

5. Kassam Z, Dubois N, Ramakrishna B, et al. Donor screening for fecal microbiota transplantation. *N Engl J Med.* 2019;381[21]:2070-2072.)

6. Edelstein C, Daw JR, Kassam Z. Seeking safe stool: Canada needs a universal donor model. *CMAJ.* 2016;188(17-18):E431-E432

7. Hu J, Torres AG. Enteropathogenic *Escherichia coli*: foe or innocent bystander? *Clin Microbiol Infect.* 2015;21(8):729-734.

8. McMichael TM, Currie DW, Clark S, et al. Epidemiology of COVID-19 in a long-term care facility in King County, Washington. *N Engl J Med.* 2020;382(21):2005-2011.

9. Allegretti JR, Kassam Z, Osman M, Budree S, Fischer M, Kelly CR. The 5D framework: a clinical primer for fecal microbiota transplantation to treat *Clostridium difficile* infection. *Gastrointest Endosc.* 2018;87(1):18-29.

10. Cammarota G, Ianiro G, Kelly CR, et al. International consensus conference on stool banking for faecal microbiota transplantation in clinical practice. *Gut.* 2019;68:2111-2121.

11. Davidovics ZH, Michail S, Nicholson MR, et al. Fecal microbiota transplantation for recurrent *Clostridium difficile* infection and other conditions in children: a joint position paper from the North American Society for Pediatric Gastroenterology, Hepatology, and Nutrition and the European Society for Pediatric Gastroenterology, Hepatology, and Nutrition. *J Pediatr Gastroenterol Nutr.* 2019;68(1):130-143.

12. Yatsunenko T, Rey FE, Manary MJ, et al. Human gut microbiome viewed across age and geography. *Nature.* 2012;486(7402):222-227.

13. US Food and Drug Administration. Important safety alert regarding use of fecal microbiota for transplantation and risk of serious adverse reactions due to transmission of multi-drug resistant organisms. https://www.fda.gov/vaccines-blood-biologics/safety-availability-biologics/important-safety-alert-regarding-use-fecal-microbiota-transplantation-and-risk-serious-adverse. Published June 13, 2019. Accessed June 13, 2020.

14. Carlson PE Jr. Regulatory considerations for fecal microbiota transplantation products. *Cell Host Microbe.* 2020;27(2):173-175.

15. Xiao F, Tang M, Zheng X, Liu Y, Li X, Shan H. Evidence for gastrointestinal infection of SARS-CoV-2. *Gastroenterology.* 2020;158(6):1831-1833.e3.

16. Ianiro G, Mullish BH, Kelly CR, et al. Screening of faecal microbiota transplant donors during the COVID-19 outbreak: suggestions for urgent updates from an international expert panel. *Lancet Gastroenterol Hepatol.* 2020;5(5):430-432.

17. Nicholson M, Alexander E, Bartlett M, Becker P, Kahn S. Fecal microbiota transplantation in pediatric *Clostridium difficile* infection, a multi-center study. *J Pediatr Gastroenterol Nutr.* 2017;65(2).

18. Moayyedi P, Surette MG, Kim PT, et al. Fecal microbiota transplantation induces remission in patients with active ulcerative colitis in a randomized controlled trial. *Gastroenterology.* 2015;149(1):102-109.e6.

19. Paramsothy S, Kamm MA, Kaakoush NO, et al. Multidonor intensive faecal microbiota transplantation for active ulcerative colitis: a randomised placebo-controlled trial. *Lancet.* 2017;389(10075):1218-1228.

7

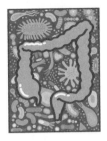

Discussion

How Do You Discuss the Risks and Benefits of Fecal Microbiota Transplantation?

Majdi Osman, MD, MPH and
Pratik Panchal, MD, MPH

Fecal microbiota transplantation (FMT) remains an investigational therapy; however, there has been significant media coverage that is likely to shape your patient's perceptions of FMT prior to counseling the patient for the procedure.[1] The widespread awareness of FMT may not have necessarily translated into a fully informed understanding of the risks, benefits, and alternatives. Sources of inaccurate information are widely available online, and patients may have preconceived ideas on the risks associated with FMT, as well as the potential benefits.[2] This lack of awareness around the risks, compounded by challenges in access, can manifest in patients seeking out do-it-yourself (DIY) treatments that present an increased hazard due to inadequate donor

Allegretti JR, Kassam Z, eds. *The 6 Ds of Fecal Microbiota Transplantation: A Primer From Decision to Discharge and Beyond* (pp 71-81).
© 2021 SLACK Incorporated.

screening and handling of material.[3] Patients may also believe that FMT could offer cures for seemingly intractable diseases beyond *Clostridioides difficile* infection (CDI) despite no current evidence or guideline recommendations supporting routine use other than for prevention of recurrent CDI.

Clear communication of the risks of FMT is crucial prior to treatment. The case reports of extended-spectrum beta-lactamase (ESBL)–producing *Escherichia coli* bacteremia following FMT highlights the importance of ensuring that risks are adequately understood.[4] Potential risks may also require some clarification with your patient to ensure the nuances are fully appreciated and to enable the patient to make an informed decision. For example, a single case report of new-onset obesity post-FMT from an overweight donor garnered significant media attention in 2015.[5] However, although weight change could be a potential risk of FMT, a more thorough analysis of 173 patients who received FMT using material from donors who were overweight, obese, and normal-weight revealed no significant weight changes post-FMT compared with their pre-CDI weight, regardless of donor weight.[6] Therefore, it is critical that when patients are initially counseled, they fully understand both the existing evidence on the risks and the potential risks that have yet to be reported.

This chapter provides you with the key points to cover when discussing FMT with your patients to support them in being fully informed ahead of undergoing treatment. This chapter will also provide advice on pre- and post-FMT care, as well as setting expectations around FMT in the context of CDI.

Informed Consent

Given the paucity of long-term safety data for FMT, it is critical to conduct and document a thorough informed consent discussion with the patient. This discussion should cover the risks and benefits of FMT material and the delivery modality, as well as any alternative treatment options, including no treatment. In addition, patients must be made aware that FMT is considered an investigational therapy, in keeping with guidance from regulatory agencies. Template informed consents are available from the Infectious Diseases Society of America[7]; however, you should make sure that the form is adapted to clearly communicate the appropriate information for your patient population and that it complies with your institution's policies. Complications related to the method of administration should be discussed separately, and patients should be given standard informed consent prior to these procedures.

Risks

In the rapidly evolving science on the microbiome, any discussion on the risks of FMT faces the challenge of navigating the nuances in clear language suitable for your patient. Approaching the discussion with your patient to understand his or her ideas, concerns, and expectations of FMT should be the initial starting point for the informed consent process.

The patient should be informed of common, mild side effects and potentially serious or life-threatening adverse events. Reactions potentially related to FMT include transient diarrhea, abdominal cramps/discomfort and nausea, fever, bloating, belching, vomiting, borborygmus, constipation, and excess flatulence.[8] These symptoms are usually self-limiting and of short duration. They may also be attributable to the delivery modality (eg, colonoscopy or upper endoscopy; Practical Pearl 7-1). There remains a paucity of prospective long-term follow-up data. Accordingly, the American Gastroenterological Association (AGA) has initiated a prospective FMT registry that will follow patients for up to 10 years. The following potential short- and long-term serious adverse events should be communicated to the patient.

Infection

Although material should have been screened for common enteric pathogens and antibiotic-resistant bacteria, there is a risk of transmission of known and unknown infectious organisms contained in the donor stool. Post-FMT bacteremia, sepsis, and fatal events may occur. Cases reported in the literature include bacteremia, cytomegalovirus (CMV) colitis, pyrexia of unknown origin, influenza B transmission, and non-CDI diarrhea (eg, norovirus).[8-10]

Immunocompromised patients should receive further counseling pre-FMT given the potential increased risk of bacteremia in this population. A multicenter retrospective study of immunocompromised patients receiving FMT to treat CDI did not report any infectious adverse events in this high-risk cohort.[11] However, the case report of ESBL *E. coli* bacteremia post-FMT in 2 immunocompromised patients highlights the risk.[4] Of note, in this case, the donor used to provide the treatments associated with these cases, administered by a hospital-based stool bank, was not screened for ESBL. Nevertheless, patients should be counseled on the risk of colonization, translocation, and infection.

Practical Pearl 7-1

What Are the Common Symptoms Your Patients May Experience Post–Fecal Microbiota Transplantation?

Transient Gastrointestinal Symptoms

24 Hours Following FMT	% Occurrence in the Literature
• Transient diarrhea	• 70%
• Abdominal pain/cramps	• 10% to 30%
• Nausea	• <5%

During the 8-Week Follow-Up Period

• Constipation	• 20%
• Excess flatulence	• 25%

Constitutional Symptoms

• Low-grade fever	• <5%

Infection Transmission Related to Fecal Microbiota Transplantation	• <1%

Sources: DeFilipp et al,[4] Lee et al,[34] Osman et al,[35] and Wang et al.[8]

Patients who are immunosuppressed and at particularly high risk of CMV or Epstein-Barr virus (EBV) infection should be counseled about the potential for additional risk of viral infections post-FMT. To date, there have only been 2 documented cases of CMV colitis in the context of FMT and no cases of EBV infection. One case report of CMV colitis occurred in a patient performing at-home, or DIY, FMT for the treatment of ulcerative colitis (UC).[12] This patient did not have CDI and used unscreened stool sourced from their child. Another small study assigned UC patients to either treatment with feces from healthy donors or to a control group receiving autologous fecal microbiota. One patient did get CMV; however, interestingly they were in the control group receiving their own autologous FMT.[13] Despite the unique features of these cases limiting their generalizability, the risks of both CMV and EBV should be clearly communicated to CMV/EBV-negative immunocompromised patients. Informed consent should also include information about the potential for transmission of severe acute respiratory syndrome coronavirus 2 via FMT, including FMT prepared from stool from donors who are asymptomatic for coronavirus 2019 (see Chapter 6: "Donor: How Do You Select and Screen Candidate Donors for Fecal Microbiota Transplantation?").

Gastrointestinal

Abdominal pain, appendicitis, peritonitis, and diverticulitis have been reported as possibly related to FMT in cases reported in the peer-reviewed literature.[8,14-17] There is a theoretical risk of small intestinal bacterial overgrowth when FMT is delivered into the upper gastrointestinal (GI) tract; however, there have been no reported cases to date.

Allergy/Anaphylaxis to Antigens in Donor Stool

Although no cases of allergy or anaphylaxis have been reported in the literature, patients should be screened for food allergies before FMT. If a patient reports a severe food allergy or anaphylaxis, he or she should be evaluated by an allergist to confirm the allergy if there is clinical uncertainty; if confirmed, one may consider using material from a patient-selected donor who has abstained from the offending agent.

Autoimmune

Rheumatoid arthritis, Sjögren's syndrome, peripheral neuropathy, and idiopathic thrombocytopenic purpura have all been reported in the peer-reviewed literature as possibly related to FMT in a case series.[18] There remains a paucity of long-term prospective follow-up evaluating the emergence of autoimmune conditions post-FMT; however, there are 2 retrospective series evaluating the long-term effects following FMT. A Finnish cohort study[19] did not detect any increased risk of autoimmune diseases compared with standard-of-care (SOC), with a mean follow-up of 3.8 years. Another cohort from the United States (N = 208) with a mean follow-up of 2.8 years identified 2 cases of psoriatic arthritis and 1 case of mastocytosis.[20]

Noninfectious Disease Transmission

There is a theoretical risk of developing diseases that may be related to donor gut microbiota. These include obesity, metabolic syndrome, neurologic disorders, psychiatric conditions, and malignancy. Persons with these known conditions should be excluded from donating stool, although a theoretical risk of acquiring these conditions and other unknown microbiome-mediated diseases after FMT remains. In the Finnish cohort,[19] there was no significant increase in cases of diabetes mellitus, neurologic diseases, malignancy, or allergies in the FMT cohort compared with those who received SOC. The cohort from the United States reported single cases of diabetes type 2, Alzheimer's dementia, and new-onset anxiety disorder during the follow-up period.[20]

Inflammatory Bowel Disease Flare

In those with underlying inflammatory bowel disease (IBD), flares have been reported in retrospective studies in which FMT was performed for CDI, with reports as high as 30%.[21] A meta-analysis revealed that among all reports of FMT performed in patients with IBD, the risk of worsening of underlying IBD was higher among the cohort receiving FMT for CDI.[22] Patients receiving FMT for the treatment of IBD had negligible rates of IBD worsening. In a prospective trial of 50 IBD patients receiving FMT for the treatment of CDI, only 2% (1/50) of patients met criteria for a de novo flare (quiescent disease at FMT and a documented increase in partial Mayo score post-FMT). Notably, the majority of patients, both UC and Crohn's disease, experienced improvement in their IBD symptoms. Risk of worsening of IBD should be discussed with your patients; however, if a patient has active IBD at the time of FMT, his or her IBD will likely still be active afterward, and further treatment plans should be discussed. At the time of writing, the large prospective AGA registry reported that among patients with 6 month follow-up, 2 patients (1%) were diagnosed with IBD.[25]

Long-Term Safety Outcomes

There is a paucity of data on the long-term safety outcomes of FMT. Therefore, a critical point to cover during your discussion is to ensure your patient fully understands that the long-term safety of FMT remains unknown. Of the available data, the long-term safety profile of FMT appears favorable; however, few prospective studies have followed up patients beyond 6 months.[18,23,24] This lack of data is especially relevant for counseling pediatric patients. Preliminary results of the real-world AGA registry (N = 259) suggest a favorable safety profile; at 6 months, new diagnoses of irritable bowel syndrome (IBS) were made in 2 patients (1%) and inflammatory bowel disease in 2 patients (1%).[25]

Procedure-Related Risks

The chosen delivery modality carries risks independent of FMT material. There have been serious adverse events reported in the peer-reviewed literature determined to be definitely related to the FMT procedure. These include aspiration after upper delivery of FMT and bowel perforation after colonoscopic delivery of FMT.[26,27] Importantly, these adverse events were related to the FMT procedure and associated with the delivery modality. Risks related to the FMT procedure should be clearly discussed with the patient, and the choice of delivery modality may depend on the patient or specific clinical situation.

Setting Expectations Following Fecal Microbiota Transplantation

Although FMT has shown promising results in randomized clinical trials and in the real-world setting of CDI, patient expectations should be calibrated appropriately during the discussion. Two points that should be discussed are treatment failure and post-infection IBS (Practical Pearl 7-2).

Treatment Failure

The potential of treatment failure should be discussed explicitly. In a 328-patient cohort, predictors of FMT failure were severe or severe-complicated CDI, inpatient status during FMT, and previous CDI-related hospitalization. With each additional hospitalization, the odds of failure increased by 43%.[28] Therefore, although FMT has been successful in clinical trials (number needed to treat = 3),[29] there is potential for treatment failure or incomplete resolution of patient's symptoms.

Post-Infection Irritable Bowel Syndrome

Patients with CDI have a high risk for developing post-infection IBS, particularly those with longer duration of CDI who might typically be assessed for FMT.[30] Up to 25% to 30% of CDI patients develop post-infection IBS. These rates appear similar in FMT patients, where rates of 28% have been observed at 8-week follow-up.[31,32] Pre-existing IBS, IBD, duration of CDI greater than 7 days, and raised body mass index have been associated with increased risk of post-infection IBS. Neither donor stool type nor delivery modality was associated with post-FMT IBS symptoms.[26-28]

Practical Pearl 7-2

Checklist for Discussing Fecal Microbiota Transplantation With Your Patient

❑ Prepare the informed consent documentation
❑ Ask about the patient's ideas, concerns, and expectations of FMT
❑ Discuss risks
  ○ Mild symptoms: Transient diarrhea, abdominal cramps/discomfort, nausea, fever, bloating, belching, vomiting, borborygmus, constipation, and excess flatulence
  ○ Infection: Life-threatening sepsis, antibiotic-resistant infections, CMV and EBV infection in the immunocompromised patient
  ○ GI
  ○ Allergy or anaphylaxis
  ○ Autoimmune
  ○ Noninfectious disease transmission
  ○ IBD flare
  ○ Unknown risk
❑ Discuss lack of evidence on long-term safety outcomes
❑ Review procedure-related risks
❑ Expectation setting
  ○ Treatment failure
  ○ Post-infection IBS
❑ Pre-FMT action items
  ○ Cleaning high-touch surfaces at home
  ○ Stop antibiotics approximately 2 days before FMT

Pre–Fecal Microbiota Transplantation Patient Education

Patients should be given clear advice on how to clean their home bathroom and high-touch surfaces before FMT to prevent ongoing exposure to spores and CDI reinfection. Specifically, patients should be advised that traditional household cleaning products are not sufficient and they should use an Environmental Protection Agency–registered disinfectant with a *C. difficile*–sporicidal label claim.[33] These agents can be any chlorine-containing cleaning agents at a concentration of at least 5000 ppm (eg, household bleach diluted with 1 part bleach to 10 parts water). Patients should take precautions in cleaning high-touch surfaces by cleaning them with at least 10 minutes of contact between a surface and the disinfectant. If a patient lives in an assisted living residence, he or she should speak to the director of the facility to ensure that the appropriate measures are taken to disinfect his or her living environment (see Chapter 9: "Discharge: How Should You Follow and Care for Patients After Fecal Microbiota Transplantation?").

Summary

A confluence of factors makes FMT a complex topic to discuss with patients. A relatively novel therapy, the emerging science of the microbiome, widespread media coverage, online forums, and a patient population that has likely failed multiple courses of antibiotics can create a challenging set of preconceived ideas, concerns, and expectations. Therefore, listening to your patient and taking time go into the nuances of the risks, benefits, and possible treatment outcomes are of great importance.

References

1. Zimmer C. Fecal transplants can be life-saving, but how? *The New York Times*. https://www.nytimes.com/2016/07/15/science/fecal-transplants-bacteria-viruses.html. Published July 15, 2016. Accessed June 16, 2020.

2. Wolf-Meyer MJ. Normal, regular, and standard: scaling the body through fecal microbial transplants. *Med Anthropol Q*. 2017;31(3):297-314.

3. Ekekezie C, Simmons S, Perler B, et al. Understanding the scope of do-it-yourself (DIY) fecal microbiota transplant (FMT). *Am J Gastroenterol*. 2018;113(suppl):S102.

4. DeFilipp Z, Bloom PP, Torres Soto M, et al. Drug-resistant *E coli* bacteremia transmitted by fecal microbiota transplant. *N Engl J Med*. 2019;381(21):2043-2050.

5. Gallagher J. Woman's stool transplant leads to "tremendous weight gain." BBC News. https://www.bbc.co.uk/news/health-31168511. Published February 7, 2015. Accessed June 16, 2020.

6. Fischer M, Kao D, Kassam Z, et al. Stool donor body mass index does not affect recipient weight after a single fecal microbiota transplantation for *Clostridium difficile* infection. *Clin Gastroenterol Hepatol*. 2018;16(8):1351-1353. doi: 10.1016/j.cgh.2017.12.007

7. Infectious Diseases Society of America. Consent for fecal microbiota transplantation (FMT). Accessed June 16, 2020. https://www.idsociety.org/globalassets/idsa/topics-of-interest/emerging-clinical-issues/fmt-consent-form.pdf

8. Wang S, Xu M, Wang W, et al. Systematic review: adverse events of fecal microbiota transplantation. *PLoS One*. 2016;11(8):e0161174.

9. Quraishi MN, Widlak M, Bhala N, et al. Systematic review with meta-analysis: the efficacy of faecal microbiota transplantation for the treatment of recurrent and refractory *Clostridium difficile* infection. *Aliment Pharmacol Ther*. 2017;46(5):479-493.

10. Baxter M, Colville A. Adverse events in faecal microbiota transplant: a review of the literature. *J Hosp Infect*. 2016;92(2):117-127.

11. Kelly CR, Ihunnah C, Fischer M, et al. Fecal microbiota transplant for treatment of *Clostridium difficile* infection in immunocompromised patients. *Am J Gastroenterol.* 2014;109(7):1065-1071.

12. Hohmann EL, Ananthakrishnan AN, Deshpande V. Case records of the Massachusetts General Hospital. Case 25-2014. A 37-year-old man with ulcerative colitis and bloody diarrhea. *N Engl J Med.* 2014;371(7):668-675.

13. Rossen NG, Fuentes S, van der Spek MJ, et al. Findings from a randomized controlled trial of fecal transplantation for patients with ulcerative colitis. *Gastroenterology.* 2015;149(1):110-118.e4.

14. Mandalia A, Kraft CS, Dhere T. Diverticulitis after fecal microbiota transplant for *C. difficile* infection. *Am J Gastroenterol.* 2014;109(12):1956-1957.

15. Kunde S, Pham A, Bonczyk S, et al. Safety, tolerability, and clinical response after fecal transplantation in children and young adults with ulcerative colitis. *J Pediatr Gastroenterol Nutr.* 2013;56(6):597-601.

16. De Leon LM, Watson JB, Kelly CR. Transient flare of ulcerative colitis after fecal microbiota transplantation for recurrent *Clostridium difficile* infection. *Clin Gastroenterol Hepatol.* 2013;11(8):1036-1038.

17. Aas J, Gessert CE, Bakken JS. Recurrent *Clostridium difficile* colitis: case series involving 18 patients treated with donor stool administered via a nasogastric tube. *Clin Infect Dis.* 2003;36(5):580-585.

18. Brandt LJ, Aroniadis OC, Mellow M, et al. Long-term follow-up of colonoscopic fecal microbiota transplant for recurrent *Clostridium difficile* infection. *Am J Gastroenterol.* 2012;107(7):1079-1087.

19. Jalanka J, Hillamaa A, Satokari R, Mattila E, Anttila V-J, Arkkila P. The long-term effects of faecal microbiota transplantation for gastrointestinal symptoms and general health in patients with recurrent *Clostridium difficile* infection. *Aliment Pharmacol Ther.* 2018;47(3):371-379.

20. Perler BK, Chen B, Phelps E, et al. Long-term efficacy and safety of fecal microbiota transplantation for treatment of recurrent *Clostridioides difficile* infection. *J Clin Gastroenterol.* 2020;54(8):701-706.

21. Fischer M, Kao D, Kelly C, et al. Fecal microbiota transplantation is safe and efficacious for recurrent or refractory *Clostridium difficile* infection in patients with inflammatory bowel disease. *Inflamm Bowel Dis.* 2016;22(10):2402-2409.

22. Qazi T, Amaratunga T, Barnes EL, et al. The risk of inflammatory bowel disease flares after fecal microbiota transplantation: systematic review and meta-analysis. *Gut Microbes.* 2017;8(6):574-588.

23. Agrawal M, Aroniadis OC, Brandt LJ, et al. The long-term efficacy and safety of fecal microbiota transplant for recurrent, severe, and complicated *Clostridium difficile* infection in 146 elderly individuals. *J Clin Gastroenterol.* 2016;50(5):403-407.

24. Nicholson M, Alexander E, Bartlett M, Becker P, Kahn S. Fecal microbiota transplantation in pediatric *Clostridium difficile* infection, a multi-center study. *J Pediatr Gastroenterol Nutr.* 2017;65(2).

25. Kelly CR, Yen EF, Grinspan AM, et al. Fecal microbiota transplant is highly effective in real-world practice: initial results from the FMT National Registry. *Gastroenterology.* 2020:S0016-5085(20)35221-5. doi:10.1053/j.gastro.2020.09.038. Epub ahead of print.

26. Obi O, Hampton D, Anderson T, Leung P, Abdul MKM, Chandra G. Fecal microbiota transplant for treatment of resistant *C. difficile* infection using a standardized protocol: a community hospital experience. *Am J Gastroenterol.* 2014;109(suppl 2):S629.

27. Baxter M, Ahmad T, Colville A, Sheridan R. Fatal aspiration pneumonia as a complication of fecal microbiota transplant. *Clin Infect Dis.* 2015;61(1):136-137.

28. Fischer M, Kao D, Mehta SR, et al. Predictors of early failure after fecal microbiota transplantation for the therapy of *Clostridium difficile* infection: a multicenter study. *Am J Gastroenterol.* 2016;111(7):1024-1031.

29. Moayyedi P, Yuan Y, Baharith H, Ford AC. Faecal microbiota transplantation for *Clostridium difficile*-associated diarrhoea: a systematic review of randomised controlled trials. *Med J Aust.* 2017;207(4):166-172.

30. Wadhwa A, Al Nahhas MF, Dierkhising RA, et al. High risk of post-infectious irritable bowel syndrome in patients with *Clostridium difficile* infection. *Aliment Pharmacol Ther.* 2016;44(6):576-582.

31. Garg S, Song Y, Han MAT, Girotra M, Fricke WF, Dutta S. 392 post-infectious irritable bowel syndrome in patients undergoing fecal microbiota transplantation for recurrent *Clostridium difficile* colitis. *Gastroenterology.* 2014;146(5 suppl 1):S83-S84.

32. Allegretti JR, Kassam Z, Sitko J, Fischer M, Chan WW. Risk factors for symptoms of post-infectious irritable bowel syndrome following fecal microbiota transplantation. *Am J Gastroenterol.* 2017;112:S655-S656.

33. United States Environmental Protection Agency. EPA's registered antimicrobial products effective against *Clostridium difficile* spores. https://www.epa.gov/sites/production/files/2020-03/documents/2020.03.04_list_k.pdf. Published March 4, 2020. Accessed June 16, 2020.

34. Lee CH, Steiner T, Petrof EO, et al. Frozen vs fresh fecal microbiota transplantation and clinical resolution of diarrhea in patients with recurrent *Clostridium difficile* infection: a randomized clinical trial. *JAMA.* 2016;315(2):142-149.

35. Osman M, O'Brien K, Stoltzner Z, et al. Safety and efficacy of fecal microbiota transplantation for recurrent Clostridium difficile infection from an international public stool bank: results from a 2050-patient multicenter cohort. *Open Forum Infect Dis.* 2016;3(suppl 1):2120.

8

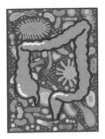

Delivery

How Do You Select the Most Appropriate Delivery Modality for Fecal Microbiota Transplantation?

Paul Feuerstadt, MD, FACG, AGAF and Neil Stollman, MD, FACP, FACG, AGAF

There are several approaches to performing a fecal microbiota transplantation (FMT), and it can be confusing to decide which approach is optimal for you and your patient. The options include administration into the upper gastrointestinal (GI) tract (eg, via upper endoscopy, nasoenteric tube, orally administered capsules) or the lower GI tract (eg, via enema, flexible sigmoidoscopy, colonoscopy; Table 8-1). Also, providers who perform FMT vary according to training, with gastroenterologists and surgeons being able to perform upper endoscopy, flexible sigmoidoscopy, and colonoscopy, and

Allegretti JR, Kassam Z, eds. *The 6 Ds of Fecal Microbiota Transplantation: A Primer From Decision to Discharge and Beyond* (pp 83-91).
© 2021 SLACK Incorporated.

Table 8-1. Advantages and Drawbacks of Delivery Modalities for Fecal Microbiota Transplantation			
	Special Training Required	Safety	Efficacy
Upper Administration			
Nasoenteric tube	X	++	++
Capsule	X	+++	+++
Lower Administration			
Enema	X	+++	+
Flexible sigmoidoscopy	√	++	+++
Colonoscopy	√	++	+++
Rating: + Good, ++ Very good, +++ Excellent.			

those trained in infectious disease or primary care being limited to the less invasive methods, such as enema, oral capsule, and nasoenteric administration.

How does one choose a modality? There is a lot to consider, and this chapter will succinctly outline the methodologies and key data supporting them to assist you in optimizing selection of the most appropriate FMT delivery modality.

Preparation Prior to Fecal Microbiota Transplantation

The ideal preparation prior to FMT is currently unknown and requires further investigation. Factors to consider include whether patients should remain on antibiotics until FMT, the timing of stoppage of antibiotics prior to FMT, and the utility of purging the bowel prior to the procedure.

Standard-of-care (SOC) antibiotics are used to treat *Clostridioides difficile* infection (CDI); however, when an FMT is indicated following SOC antibiotics, the course of antibiotics is often extended up until the time of FMT to prevent a subsequent recurrence prior to FMT (Practical Pearl 8-1). However, this is not a data-supported method. The

Practical Pearl 8-1

How Do You Prepare Your Patient for a Fecal Microbiota Transplantation?

- Prior to the day of the FMT, patients should be advised to hold their SOC antibiotic (eg, vancomycin). Typically, it is held from 1 to 3 days prior to FMT.
  - ○ Clinical tip: If administering via colonoscopy, have patients take their last doses the day before the bowel lavage. The preparation will help to wash out any residual vancomycin.
- Standard bowel lavage is performed the day before FMT by colonoscopy. This is to assist with luminal visualization and also potentially remove any residual antibiotics and possibly spores.
  - ○ Bowel preparation is generally not given before upper GI tract delivery, including capsules.

ideal antibiotic choice and optimal length of therapy preceding FMT remain unknown. In practice, most clinicians performing FMT continue to administer SOC antibiotics until the FMT procedure can be set up logistically. At high-volume FMT centers, this can often be organized in a few days, but at lower-volume centers, this might take a week if on-demand shipping from a stool bank is the source of the material, or it may be even longer if the clinicians are using a patient-selected model. Given the recurrent nature of CDI and the risks off antibiotics, the most ethical, and practical, intervention seems to be to continue suppressive therapy until FMT can be performed.

The time to stop SOC antibiotics prior to FMT is a matter of debate as well. Most practitioners will stop these therapies 1 to 3 days prior to the procedure. This is believed to be a reasonable window allowing sufficient time to clear the majority of the antimicrobial! from the patient's system while still limiting the rapid reproliferation of *C. difficile* off treatment. Further investigation is needed to clarify this issue.

Another area of debate with limited data involves whether a bowel lavage enhances the efficacy of FMT. A bowel preparation theoretically purges the majority of the original deficient microbiota from the patient prior to the FMT, allowing the newly introduced microbiota a more favorable environment for engraftment. In most practices, purging enemas are given prior to FMT via flexible sigmoidoscopy, and full bowel purge is only performed prior to colonoscopic FMT. Most providers do not give a bowel lavage prior to nasoenteric infusions or capsule or enema administration.

Upper Gastrointestinal Tract Administration

There are 2 main methods for FMT delivery via the upper GI tract: nasoenteric infusion and orally administered capsules. A naso-enteric infusion is a procedure where a nasogastric, nasoduodenal, or nasojejunal tube is passed into the patient and FMT material is infused. The first prospective randomized clinical trial of patients with recurrent CDI (rCDI) reporting superiority of FMT to a standard antibiotic course with vancomycin, used FMT via nasoduodenal tube infusion.[1] This prospective study was important because it showed that, in addition to significantly higher rates of clinical cure of CDI, the recipient's micro-biota diversity was restored following FMT.[1] Despite this method's efficacy and its visibility in such an important trial, it has significant drawbacks given the discomforts of passage of a nasoenteric tube, the patient visualizing FMT material being passed into their digestive tract, and risks of aspiration of the material. On the other hand, this modal-ity can be performed by most practitioners, so this remains a viable option in some centers.

It is worth noting that there are different risk profiles to naso-gastric (the most logistically feasible) vs nasoduodenal or nasojejunal tubes. Due to the administration of the FMT material in the pre-pyloric location, the risk of aspiration is higher using a nasogastric tube than nasoduodenal or nasojejunal tubes, which are both post-pyloric. Newer nasoduodenal/nasojejunal systems may permit visualization, and these are more commonly used in Europe. That said, from a patient perspective, perception studies suggest that patients would prefer not to undergo an FMT via nasoenteric tube administration.[2]

An easier and more palatable method of FMT is via orally admin-istered capsules, which can be provided by all practitioners. With this method, FMT material is directly enclosed in a coated capsule, which is swallowed by the patient, either in one sitting or over the course of several days. Depending on the capsule formulation, prior to tak-ing the capsules some patients are advised to take acid suppressive medications, such as proton-pump inhibitors. This is done to theo-retically minimize capsule breakdown in the acidic environment of the stomach, thereby minimizing degradation of the FMT material in the proximal digestive tract. There is no high-quality data to support or refute this approach; however, the need may be related of the specific capsule coating. Youngster et al[3] published data from an open-label pilot study (N = 20) using orally administered capsules (15 capsules on 2 consecutive days) showing that with 1 or 2 courses, patients with rCDI had an overall clinical cure rate of 90%, without any serious related adverse events. Other studies have also shown reasonable efficacy and safety profiles with capsule FMT, and given the ease of administration and patient preference, we suspect it will be the most commonly used modality in the future.

In outlining FMT administration techniques of the upper GI tract, we have presented data for CDI, in which the goal is to reconstitute the depleted colonic microbiota. The upper administrative techniques will commonly distribute FMT material into the small bowel in addition to the large bowel. It has been speculated that this may be associated with greater rates of post-procedure small intestinal bacterial overgrowth and gas/bloat symptoms; however, Allegretti et al[4,5] conducted a large cohort study that suggests this may not be a concern. In one study comparing capsules designed to release in the colon with others starting release in the stomach, clinical cure rates for CDI were similar between both groups, but colonic engraftment of the donor stool was higher in the capsules with colonic release.[6] Although underpowered, this study suggests there may be utility in precision targeting of FMT material.

There are still many unanswered questions regarding FMT by upper GI tract, including the ideal dose/dose regimen (eg, the number of capsules, volume of stool infused via nasoenteric tube, and concentration of microbial species administered); whether lyophilized, frozen, or fresh capsule formulations are optimal; whether single- or multi-day administration is preferable; and the role, if any, of adjunctive acid suppression.

Lower Gastrointestinal Tract Administration

There are 3 main methods of lower GI tract administration, including enema, flexible sigmoidoscopy, and colonoscopy. Enema administration can be performed in the office setting, where a patient is placed in left lateral decubitus position and a flexible catheter is inserted into the rectum, through which the FMT material is then infused. This method was first shown to be safe and effective in patients with CDI by Kassam et al[7,8] using a retention enema. In a follow-up study of retention enema FMT for CDI, Lee et al[9] compared frozen and thawed stool with freshly donated FMT material and reported that frozen was noninferior to fresh. The similar efficacy supports the efficient process of stool banks freezing and shipping samples to centers, sparing them the expensive and onerous screening process. However, it should be noted that the efficacy after a single FMT via enema in both groups was low (62.7% frozen vs 62.1% fresh). For CDI, FMT via enema remains an option, but this also requires more investigation to clarify the volume of donor material required, the minimum duration that the enema should be retained, and whether a single enema is sufficient. Enemas also seem safe with a theoretical risk for perforation, but this has yet to be reported, and this method allows for direct administration of the microbiota to the colon.

Colonoscopy and flexible sigmoidoscopy are procedures where a flexible tube with a fiber-optic camera at the tip is passed into the colon. This technique is most commonly used to inspect the lining of the colon and assess for pathology. When it is being used for FMT, the scope is either passed about one-third of the length of the colon (eg, flexible sigmoidoscopy) or the entire length of the large bowel (eg, colonoscopy). Prior to flexible sigmoidoscopy, a saline enema is usually administered to cleanse the distal colon that will be inspected. Before a colonoscopy, a large-volume purge of the colonic contents is required. For FMT, at the time when the endoscope has reached its most proximal point in the bowel, FMT material is passed through the endoscope directly into the bowel lumen. This is commonly given either as a single administration in the most proximal area of bowel reached (ie, terminal ileum or cecum) or in segments, including the cecum and ascending and transverse colon. In the segmental approach, it is less commonly distributed in the left colon given that the material from the proximal large bowel will traverse this region, distributing the transplanted material.

There are multiple studies supporting the safety and efficacy for FMT by colonoscopy in those with rCDI and administration of fresh stool is similar to frozen and thawed.[10,11] Some providers administer loperamide 2 to 4 mg either just prior to or following the FMT by colonoscopy, in an effort to increase the duration of retention of the transplanted material and enhance the likelihood of engraftment. There are insufficient data to support or refute this intervention. As with all methods of FMT, there are limitations to using colonoscopy/flexible sigmoidoscopy, including the invasive nature of the procedures and that colonoscopy most commonly requires monitored anesthesia care for sedation. There are also risks associated with endoscopic interventions, including risks of anesthesia and standard endoscopic risks, such as bleeding, infection, and perforation. In the setting of FMT, the benefits of the therapy frequently outweigh the risks, but the clinician needs to consider these factors when choosing a modality.

Unanswered questions include the optimal dose/dose regimen, the ideal locations within the colon the material should be administered, whether loperamide usage is beneficial, and whether there is a threshold of time following the FMT, prior to passage of stool from the patient, that optimizes efficacy.

Efficacies of the Various Modalities

In the first meta-analysis performed considering the efficacy of FMT in patients with rCDI, Kassam et al[10] assessed 11 case series including 273 patients and reported that FMT was 89% effective at preventing CDI recurrence. In addition, overall, lower administration was more effective than upper modalities.[10] Quraishi et al[11] performed a more recent meta-analysis that considered 37 studies, including numerous case series and 7 randomized clinical trials (N = 1973). This meta-analysis once again showed that lower administration (92% to 97%) was more efficacious than upper modalities (82% to 94%; $P = .02$).[11] Given the colonic involvement of CDI, the superior efficacy of lower administration techniques is logical and reinforced by these data.

Some studies have compared modalities head-to-head in patients with CDI. Kao et al[12] conducted a randomized clinical trial (N = 116) that compared FMT via frozen oral capsules vs frozen FMT material delivered via colonoscopy. In this study, capsule administration (96.2%) was noninferior to colonoscopy (96.2%), with no related serious adverse events.[12] In another study that compared lyophilized FMT capsules vs FMT enema with frozen FMT material, capsules (84%) yielded similar efficacy to the enema treatment (88%; $P = .76$).[13]

Summary

We have many options to deliver FMT to patients, but quite a bit of research is still needed to identify the specifics of delivery. The choice of the most appropriate should be driven in part by the options available to the provider and, of course, the preferences of the well-informed patient. Meta-analyses support lower GI administration techniques being modestly more efficacious than upper, but head-to-head trials show similar efficacies between FMT by capsule and colonoscopy. Less invasive methods clinically seem to be best from a patient care prospective and universal ability of providers to administer the FMT. Given this, capsules may end up being the most widely adopted. As a clinician, it is probably best to follow this axiom to choose which FMT modality is best for your patient population (Practical Pearl 8-2).

Practical Pearl 8-2

How Do You Select the Right Delivery Modality for Your Patient?

There are many considerations when deciding on the appropriate delivery modality for your patients. Here are a few practical points to keep in mind:

- Dysphagia or significant GI motility disorders: If a patient has ongoing dysphagia or any difficulty swallowing pills, FMT by capsule should be avoided to minimize aspiration risk. Additionally, a patient with a significant GI motility disorder, such as gastroparesis, should also avoid FMT capsules.
- Major comorbidities: If a patient has significant comorbidities that would make sedation unsafe (eg, significant cardiorespiratory disease), consider FMT by capsule (or possibly enema) as opposed to colonoscopy.
- Colostomy: In a patient with a colostomy, endoscopic administration can be performed via the stoma.
- Potential GI pathology: If there is concern about underlying luminal pathology, colonoscopy is preferred for mucosal assessment and biopsy.
- Patient-centric: The selection of a delivery modality should always involve a conversation with the patient regarding his or her preferences if no contraindications are present.

References

1. van Nood E, Vrieze A, Nieuwdorp M, et al. Duodenal infusion of donor feces for recurrent Clostridium difficile. N Engl J Med. 2013;368(5):407-415.
2. Zipursky JS, Sidorsky TI, Freedman CA, Sidorsky MN, Kirkland KB. Patient attitudes toward the use of fecal microbiota transplantation in the treatment of recurrent Clostridium difficile infection. Clin Infect Dis. 2012;55(12):1652-1658.
3. Youngster I, Russell GH, Pindar C, Ziv-Baran T, Sauk J, Hohmann EL. Oral, capsulized, frozen fecal microbiota transplantation for relapsing Clostridium difficile infection. JAMA. 2014;312(17):1772-1778.
4. Allegretti JR, Kassam Z, Fischer M, Kelly C, Chan WW. Risk factors for gastrointestinal symptoms following successful eradication of Clostridium difficile by fecal microbiota transplantation (FMT). J Clin Gastroenterol. 2019;53(9):e405-e408.
5. Allegretti JR, Kassam Z, Chan WW. Small intestinal bacterial overgrowth: should screening be included in the pre-fecal microbiota transplantation evaluation? Dig Dis Sci. 2018;63(1):193-197.

6. Allegretti JR, Fischer M, Sagi SV, et al. Fecal microbiota transplantation capsules with targeted colonic versus gastric delivery in recurrent *Clostridium difficile* infection: a comparative cohort analysis of high and lose dose. *Dig Dis Sci.* 2019;64(6):1672-1678.

7. Kassam Z, Hundal R, Marshall JK, Lee CH. Fecal transplant via retention enema for refractory or recurrent *Clostridium difficile* infection. *Arch Intern Med.* 2012;172(2):191-193.

8. Lee CH, Belanger JE, Kassam Z, et al. The outcome and long-term follow-up of 94 patients with recurrent and refractory *Clostridium difficile* infection using single to multiple fecal microbiota transplantation via retention enema. *Eur J Clin Microbiol Infect Dis.* 2014;33(8):1425-1428.

9. Lee CH, Steiner T, Petrof EO, et al. Frozen vs fresh fecal microbiota transplantation and clinical resolution of diarrhea in patients with recurrent *Clostridium difficile* infection: a randomized clinical trial. *JAMA.* 2016;315(2):142-149.

10. Kassam Z, Lee CH, Yuan Y, Hunt RH. Fecal microbiota transplantation for *Clostridium difficile* infection: systematic review and meta-analysis. *Am J Gastroenterol.* 2013;108(4):500-508.

11. Quraishi MN, Widlak M, Bhala N, et al. Systematic review with meta-analysis: the efficacy of faecal microbiota transplantation for the treatment of recurrent and refractory *Clostridium difficile* infection. *Aliment Pharmacol Ther.* 2017;46(5):479-493.

12. Kao D, Roach B, Silva M, et al. Effect of oral capsule- vs colonoscopy-delivered fecal microbiota transplantation on recurrent *Clostridium difficile* infection: a randomized clinical trial. *JAMA.* 2017;318(20):1985-1993.

13. Jiang ZD, Jenq RR, Ajami NJ, et al. Safety and preliminary efficacy of orally administered lyophilized fecal microbiota product compared with frozen product given by enema for recurrent *Clostridium difficile* infection: a randomized clinical trial. *PLoS One.* 2018;13(11):e0205064.

9

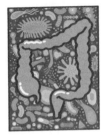

Discharge
How Should You Follow and Care for Patients After Fecal Microbiota Transplantation?

Lauren Tal Grinspan, MD, PhD and Ari M. Grinspan, MD

Now that the patient has received a fecal microbiota transplantation (FMT), it is important to discuss the discharge plan. There are a number of considerations for the patient and physician. The physician should let the patient know what possible symptoms to expect and when to follow up. The physician should know how to address questions and concerns from patients, to know when to reassure or when to be concerned. Physicians should know what diagnostic evaluation to perform and when, as well as have a contingency plan in place in case of FMT failure. This chapter will review household disinfection,

Allegretti JR, Kassam Z, eds. *The 6 Ds of Fecal Microbiota Transplantation: A Primer From Decision to Discharge and Beyond* (pp 93-102).
© 2021 SLACK Incorporated.

antibiotic stewardship, mitigating risk factors for recurrent *Clostridioides difficile* infection (rCDI), and how to manage symptoms post-FMT.

Household Disinfection

The patient's home should be disinfected, ideally on the day of FMT when the patient is out of the house. Spores are resistant to common cleaners. Therefore, we recommend using an Environmental Protection Agency–registered disinfectant with a *C. difficile*–sporicidal label claim (household bleach or a powerful chlorine agent).[1] We suggest any chlorine-containing cleaning agent with at least a concentration of 5000 ppm (eg, household bleach diluted with 1 part bleach to 10 parts water). For effective removal of these spores, one should scrub any high-touch surfaces, including toilets, faucets, showers, and doorknobs, for at least 10 minutes.[2] Additionally, we recommend washing of linens using a chlorine bleach and laundry soap at hot water temperature cycles. Patients or caregivers of patients who live in assisted living facilities should contact the facility director to ensure appropriate disinfection.

Antibiotic Stewardship

Long-term CDI recurrence rates are low after successful FMT. Mamo et al[3] reported that 82% of patients had no CDI recurrence at 22 months following FMT; however, patients who had rCDI were more commonly exposed to antibiotics than the non-rCDI group.[3] Early antibiotic use within 8 weeks of FMT has been shown to nearly triple the rate of FMT failure (27.6% vs 11.3%, $P = .01$).[4] These studies highlight the importance of antibiotic stewardship, especially in patients following FMT. Patients should be counseled on 3 important facets.[5] First, patients should be advised to avoid unnecessary antibiotics (eg, viral upper respiratory tract infection, asymptomatic bacteriuria). Second, if antibiotics are necessary, patients should be counseled about narrowing the spectrum of antibiotic, if possible, in coordination with their infectious disease specialist. Finally, the route of administration should be taken into consideration. For example, intramuscular gentamicin, which is gut microbiome sparing, has been used for the treatment of urinary tract infection (UTI) has been reported in patients with a history of rCDI to avoid the negative impact of fluoroquinolones on gut microbiome (Practical Pearl 9-1).[6]

Given the increased risk of CDI recurrence in the setting of systemic antibiotics, several groups have assessed the efficacy of CDI prophylaxis. A retrospective cohort study of patients with history of CDI in

Practical Pearl 9-1

Gut Microbiome–Sparing Antibiotic for Urinary Tract Infection

- UTIs are frequent among older adults, particularly females, who are also at risk for CDI.
- Fluoroquinolones are frequently used to treat UTIs; however, they have a negative impact on the gut microbiome and put patients at risk for a CDI recurrence.
- An example of an outpatient treatment protocol using a gut microbiome–sparing antibiotic for an uncomplicated UTIs that has been reported includes:
  - Clinical evaluation of the UTI, including documentation of infection by urinalysis and culture; rule out asymptomatic bacteriuria
  - Gentamicin administered intramuscularly at 160 mg on day 1 (2 injections in separate sites) and single 80-mg injections on days 2 and 3.
  - Intravenous infusion of gentamicin with the same dosing schedule could be offered as an alternative. A pharmacist should be consulted for dosage adjustment if a patient had an estimated glomerular filtration rate < 40 mL/min/1.73 m².

Source: Staley et al.[6]

the previous 90 days who were then exposed to non-CDI antibiotics showed that patients with 2 or more episodes of prior CDI in the past 6 to 12 months had a lower rate of CDI when receiving prophylactic CDI antibiotics (mostly vancomycin) concomitantly.[7] A more recent multicenter retrospective study showed that non-CDI antibiotic use after successful FMT significantly increases risk of rCDI.[8] These patients are more than 8 times more likely to develop CDI if they are receiving a systemic antibiotic after 8 weeks post-FMT. Interestingly, CDI antibiotic prophylaxis was not found to be protective in this cohort.[8] The most recent Infectious Diseases Society of America (IDSA) guidelines from 2018 have no recommendations regarding secondary prophylaxis for CDI. However, they state that "if the decision is to institute CDI prevention agents, it may be prudent to administer low doses of vancomycin or fidaxomicin (eg, 125 mg or 200 mg, respectively, once daily) while systemic antibiotics are administered."[9]

We recommend, if possible, avoiding antibiotics after FMT and certainly within the first 8 weeks because this is associated with treatment failure.[4] This includes avoiding elective surgeries and dental work that may necessitate antibiotic use. Overall, based on the lack of evidence, we do not recommend routine use of prophylactic CDI antibiotics if systemic antibiotics need to be used post-FMT.

Recurrent Symptoms

Gastrointestinal (GI) symptoms and altered bowel habits after FMT are common and include constipation, bloating, and loose stool. According to a prospective cohort study comparing rCDI patients who underwent FMT by either colonoscopy or capsules using patient-selected donor stool or universal stool bank donor stool, the factors associated with increased GI symptoms include younger age, baseline history of irritable bowel syndrome (IBS) and preexisting inflammatory bowel disease (IBD).[10] Symptoms were not related to donor type or mode of delivery.

If recurrent or new GI symptoms occur after FMT, a broad differential should be considered based on clinical presentation. This includes non-CDI acute gastroenteritis, post-infection IBS, bile salt malabsorption, microscopic colitis, post-diarrhea lactase deficiency, small intestinal bacterial overgrowth, IBD, antibiotic-associated diarrhea, and rCDI. Figure 9-1 provides a clinical algorithm for evaluation of GI symptoms following FMT.

There have been concerns about increased IBD flares following FMT, and 4 retrospective studies have shown variable flare rates ranging from 18% to 54% after FMT.[11-15] The ICON study is the first prospective study of patients with IBD who undergo FMT for rCDI and shows 92% efficacy in this population.[16] Importantly, only 1 patient developed a de novo IBD flare (defined as a patient with inactive disease at the time of FMT, with worsening of IBD clinical scores by week 12).[16] This prospective study provides reassurance to practitioners that the clinical outcomes of FMT in the IBD population appear similar to a non-IBD cohort. We recommend that practitioners continue to follow this specific population closely and stress the importance of treating the underlying IBD appropriately.

Post-infection IBS can occur in nearly 30% of patients with CDI.[17] This is a remarkably common entity and is frequently seen in clinical practice. Typically, post-infection IBS is mild, with altered bowel symptoms and crampy abdominal pain and is worse with food intake. Patients commonly report that they feel "different" from their baseline but symptoms are usually not as severe as their prior CDI symptoms. Educating patients that they may experience these symptoms is paramount, and frequent reassurance is key. A limited evaluation may be warranted to rule out infection and inflammation and to assuage

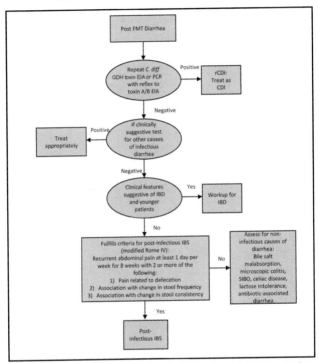

Figure 9-1. Diarrhea post–fecal microbiota transplantation workup. (toxin EIA = toxin enzyme immunoassay; GDH = glutamate dehydrogenase; PCR = polymerase chain reaction; SIBO = small intestinal bacterial overgrowth.) (Adapted from Allegretti et al.[5])

patients. Commonly, *C. difficile* testing (PCR or GDH with reflex to toxin EIA) and calprotectin are the first-line diagnostic tools. Normal results should provide reassurance to both provider and patient. Focusing on dietary modifications, including limiting dairy, fat, and sugar intake, can be helpful. There are a minority of patients who will have more severe symptoms after FMT. If symptoms are diarrhea predominant, stool testing should be pursued to rule out infection and inflammation. Diagnostic colonoscopy, imaging, and breath testing may be warranted depending on the clinical scenario (see Figure 9-1).

Fecal Microbiota Transplantation Follow-Up

After discharge, it is important to ensure close follow-up to identify FMT failure and adverse events. Additionally, patients should be counseled on when to be most alert to symptoms. An observational study looking at primary nonresponders (within 1 week), early secondary nonresponders (between weeks 1 and 4), and late secondary nonresponders (between weeks 4 and 8) found that 86% of nonresponders fail by week 4, and there are few late secondary nonresponders (Figure 9-2).[18] Accordingly, we recommend a set schedule for follow-up to identify FMT failure or adverse events that leverages this natural history. We recommend calling patients 1 week after FMT to assess for primary nonresponse and to assess at week 4 for early secondary nonresponse. Additionally, we recommend an office visit 8 weeks after FMT. If there is no recurrence, the patient can be considered clinically cured. We do not recommend testing for cure. *C. difficile* testing should only occur during the follow-up period in the setting of diarrheal symptoms. There is a low asymptomatic carriage rate post-FMT of 3% after 4 weeks.[19] As described earlier, positive stool CDI test result in the setting of an asymptomatic patient is clinically irrelevant and does not warrant treatment.

FMT failure should be considered if symptoms resemble prior episodes of CDI. In this setting, CDI testing should not be conducted unless patients are experiencing 3 or more unformed stools per day for 2 or more days, or in the case that there are other systemic symptoms suggestive of CDI.[5] To test for CDI recurrence after FMT, a 2-step approach is recommended by the European Society of Clinical Microbiology and Infectious Diseases and IDSA guidelines: initially with GDH toxin EIA or PCR testing, followed by toxin EIA for toxin A/B.[20]

If patients develop confirmed rCDI after FMT, there are several treatment strategies. All patients should be restarted on standard-of-care antibiotics. A second FMT can be performed, which has been shown to be effective with high secondary cure rates.[21-24] Other treatment options include prolonged vancomycin taper, chronic vancomycin suppression with once-daily dosing, fidaxomicin taper, and bezlotoxumab. The decision on which treatment strategy to use should be individualized based on the patient and underlying comorbidities. We recommend repeat FMT via colonoscopy, especially if the first FMT was performed via a different delivery method. In older, frail, or homebound patients, it is reasonable to consider chronic vancomycin suppression with once-daily dosing. There is minimal systemic

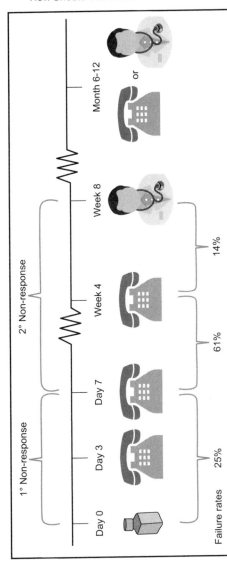

Figure 9-2. Post–fecal microbiota transplantation follow up. Phone call within 1 week to assess for primary non-response and adverse events. Phone call at 4 weeks to assess for early secondary non-response, and an office visit at week 8 to assess for new or ongoing symptoms. Phone call or visit at 6 to 12 months to assess for long-term response or adverse events.[18]

absorption and few adverse events with this strategy. Bezlotoxumab has been shown to reduce absolute risk of rCDI by 10% in average-risk patients, but reports suggest it may to be more effective in higher-risk populations (eg, older adults, immunosuppressed, renal failure), with a number needed to treat of 6 to 8.[25] However, bezlotoxumab should be avoided in patients with class 3 or 4 congestive heart failure. Although there is no clinical guideline where to position bezlotoxumab in the treatment algorithm of rCDI, we recommend considering its use after failing FMT. There are no data on combining FMT with bezlotoxumab, but there is an upcoming trial that will be exploring this option in an IBD-with-CDI population (NCT03829475).

Summary

The major goals after discharge from FMT are preventing reinfection and monitoring for treatment failure. Reinfection can be minimized through careful household disinfection and antibiotic stewardship. Although failure of FMT is uncommon, it is important to have a follow-up system in place to quickly identify those patients who have not cleared the infection. Additionally, patients and physicians should be aware of symptoms that may develop after FMT. When symptoms do occur after FMT, physicians must know when to be worried about CDI but must also be cognizant of the differential diagnosis, notably post-infection IBS. It is critical for the physician to understand when and how to perform CDI testing in the post-FMT period and the various options that are available to manage treatment failure (Practical Pearl 9-2).

References

1. United States Environmental Protection Agency. EPA's registered antimicrobial products effective against *Clostridium difficile* spores. https://www.epa.gov/sites/production/files/2020-03/documents/2020.03.04_list_k.pdf. Published March 4, 2020. Accessed June 16, 2020.
2. OpenBiome. Care after your fecal transplant. Accessed June 18, 2020. https://www.openbiome.org/patient-support
3. Mamo Y, Woodworth MH, Wang T, Dhere T, Kraft CS. Durability and long-term clinical outcomes of fecal microbiota transplant treatment in patients with recurrent *Clostridium difficile* infection. *Clin Infect Dis.* 2018;66(11):1705-1711.
4. Allegretti JR, Kao D, Sitko J, Fischer M, Kassam Z. Early antibiotic use after fecal microbiota transplantation increases risk of treatment failure. *Clin Infect Dis.* 2018;66(1):134-135.
5. Allegretti JR, Kassam Z, Osman M, Budree S, Fischer M, Kelly CR. The 5D framework: a clinical primer for fecal microbiota transplantation to treat *Clostridium difficile* infection. *Gastrointest Endosc.* 2018;87(1):18-29.

Practical Pearl 9-2

Consideration Prior to Discharging Your Patient Post–Fecal Microbiota Transplantation

- Remind your patient to not resume CDI antibiotics.
- Clean high-touch surface areas with a sporicidal cleaning agent.
- Avoid future unnecessary antibiotic use.
  - Tip: Providing a patient with a wallet card stating that he or she has had rCDI and an FMT is a useful patient empowerment tool that he or she can show physicians/pharmacists/dentists.
- Monitor for diarrhea symptoms over the next 8 weeks.
  - Counsel regarding transient GI symptoms.
- Let patient know about follow-up calls at weeks 1 and 4 post-FMT.
- Arrange follow-up visit after 8 weeks post-FMT.
- Review warning signs or reasons to return to the emergency department/hospital:
  - High fever
  - Severe abdominal pain
  - Bloody stools

6. Staley C, Vaughn BP, Graiziger CT, Sadowsky MJ, Khoruts A. Gut-sparing treatment of urinary tract infection in patients at high risk of *Clostridium difficile* infection. *J Antimicrob Chemother.* 2017;72(2):522-528.

7. Carignan A, Poulin S, Martin P, et al. Efficacy of secondary prophylaxis with vancomycin for preventing recurrent *Clostridium difficile* infections. *Am J Gastroenterol.* 2016;111(12):1834-1840.

8. Allegretti JR, Kao D, Phelps E, et al. Risk of *Clostridium difficile* infection with systemic antimicrobial therapy following successful fecal microbiota transplant: should we recommend anti-*Clostridium difficile* antibiotic prophylaxis? *Dig Dis Sci.* 2019;64(6):1668-1671.

9. McDonald LC, Gerding DN, Johnson S, et al. Clinical practice guidelines for *Clostridium difficile* infection in adults and children: 2017 update by the Infectious Diseases Society of America (IDSA) and Society for Healthcare Epidemiology of America (SHEA). *Clin Infect Dis.* 2018;66(7):987-994.

10. Allegretti JR, Kassam Z, Fischer M, Kelly C, Chan WW. Risk factors for gastrointestinal symptoms following successful eradication of *Clostridium difficile* by fecal microbiota transplantation (FMT). *J Clin Gastroenterol.* 2019;53(9):e405-e408.

11. Khoruts A, Rank KM, Newman KM, et al. Inflammatory bowel disease affects the outcome of fecal microbiota transplantation for recurrent *Clostridium difficile* infection. *Clin Gastroenterol Hepatol.* 2016;14(10):1433-1438.

12. Newman KM, Rank KM, Vaughn BP, Khoruts A. Treatment of recurrent *Clostridium difficile* infection using fecal microbiota transplantation in patients with inflammatory bowel disease. *Gut Microbes.* 2017;8(3):303-309.

13. Fischer M, Kao D, Kelly C, et al. Fecal microbiota transplantation is safe and efficacious for recurrent or refractory *Clostridium difficile* infection in patients with inflammatory bowel disease. *Inflamm Bowel Dis.* 2016;22(10):2402-2409.

14. Chin SM, Sauk J, Mahabamunuge J, Kaplan JL, Hohmann EL, Khalili H. Fecal microbiota transplantation for recurrent *Clostridium difficile* infection in patients with inflammatory bowel disease: a single-center experience. *Clin Gastroenterol Hepatol.* 2017;15(4):597-599.

15. Hirten RP, Grinspan A, Fu SC, et al. Microbial engraftment and efficacy of fecal microbiota transplant for *Clostridium difficile* in patients with and without inflammatory bowel disease. *Inflamm Bowel Dis.* 2019;25(6):969-979.

16. Allegretti JR, Hurtado J, Carrellas M, et al. The ICON Study: inflammatory bowel disease and recurrent *Clostridium difficile* infection: outcomes after fecal microbiota transplantation. *Gastroenterology.* 2019;156(6):S-2-S-3.

17. Wadhwa A, Al Nahhas MF, Dierkhising RA, et al. High risk of post-infectious irritable bowel syndrome in patients with *Clostridium difficile* infection. *Aliment Pharmacol Ther.* 2016;44(6):576-582.

18. Allegretti JR, Allegretti AS, Phelps E, Xu H, Fischer M, Kassam Z. Classifying fecal microbiota transplantation failure: an observational study examining timing and characteristics of fecal microbiota transplantation failures. *Clin Gastroenterol Hepatol.* 2018;16(11):1832-1833.

19. Allegretti JR, Allegretti AS, Phelps E, Xu H, Kassam Z, Fischer M. Asymptomatic *Clostridium difficile* carriage rate post-fecal microbiota transplant is low: a prospective clinical and stool assessment. *Clin Microbiol Infect.* 2018;24(7):780.e1-780.e3.

20. Crobach MJ, Planche T, Eckert C, et al. European Society of Clinical Microbiology and Infectious Diseases: update of the diagnostic guidance document for *Clostridium difficile* infection. *Clin Microbiol Infect.* 2016;22(suppl 4):S63-S81.

21. Aroniadis OC, Brandt LJ, Greenberg A, et al. Long-term follow-up study of fecal microbiota transplantation for severe and/or complicated *Clostridium difficile* infection: a multicenter experience. *J Clin Gastroenterol.* 2016;50(5):398-402.

22. Brandt LJ, Aroniadis OC, Mellow M, et al. Long-term follow-up of colonoscopic fecal microbiota transplant for recurrent *Clostridium difficile* infection. *Am J Gastroenterol.* 2012;107(7):1079-1087.

23. Kelly CR, Khoruts A, Staley C, et al. Effect of fecal microbiota transplantation on recurrence in multiply recurrent *Clostridium difficile* infection: a randomized trial. *Ann Intern Med.* 2016;165(9):609-616.

24. Satokari R, Mattila E, Kainulainen V, Arkkila PE. Simple faecal preparation and efficacy of frozen inoculum in faecal microbiota transplantation for recurrent *Clostridium difficile* infection—an observational cohort study. *Aliment Pharmacol Ther.* 2015;41(1):46-53.

25. Wilcox MH, Gerding DN, Poxton IR, et al. Bezlotoxumab for prevention of recurrent *Clostridium difficile* infection. *N Engl J Med.* 2017;376(4):305-317.

10

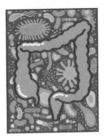

Discovery
Emerging Indications

Jessica R. Allegretti, MD, MPH and
Zain Kassam, MD, MPH

For many years, peptic ulcers were thought to be related to stress and lifestyle factors. Dr. Barry Marshall and Dr. Robin Warren's groundbreaking work suggested a radical idea: that a microbe, *Helicobacter pylori*, played a major role in many peptic ulcers.[1] There were significant headwinds to the proposal that microbes may be the underlying cause. In fact, Marshall and Warren's original *H. pylori* research abstract in 1983 was not accepted for presentation. A few years later, they received the Nobel Prize. This story highlights the power of microbes and the concept that the microbiome may have an impact on diseases that do not seem intuitive, both in the GI tract and beyond.

Allegretti JR, Kassam Z, eds. *The 6 Ds of Fecal Microbiota Transplantation: A Primer From Decision to Discharge and Beyond* (pp 103-175).
© 2021 SLACK Incorporated.

Although the majority of data and clinical experience for FMT are for the prevention of recurrent *Clostridioides difficile* infection (rCDI), there has been a rapid growth in translational research examining the role of the microbiome in many diseases and preliminary investigation of fecal microbiota transplantation (FMT) in a number of microbiome-mediated clinical conditions. The following sections serve as a current state-of-the-field to outline the most promising indication for FMT and microbiome therapies. In the pages ahead, we outline the evidence for other CDI phenotypes, such as primary CDI and severe and fulminant disease, and also navigate the data for inflammatory bowel disease (IBD) and irritable bowel syndrome (IBS). Additionally, we move beyond the GI tract and explore the gut–liver axis, gut–brain axis, decolonization of antibiotic-resistant bacteria, and even the role of FMT for metabolic conditions, such as obesity. This overview represents the tip of the proverbial iceberg as scientists and physicians continue to explore this nascent field.

FMT for these conditions is still investigational. Data will continue to emerge and potentially transform our approach to patients suffering from microbiome-mediated diseases.

Reference

1. Pincock S. Nobel Prize winners Robin Warren and Barry Marshall. *Lancet.* 2005;366(945). doi:10.1016/S0140-6736(05)67587-3

10.1

Other *Clostridioides difficile* Indications

10.1.1 The Role of Fecal Microbiota Transplantation in the Treatment of Primary *Clostridioides difficile* Infection

Alexander Khoruts, MD

Given the evidence of FMT for recurrent *Clostridium difficile* infection (rCDI; previously recurrent *Clostridium difficile* infection),[1] there has been interest in the use of FMT for primary CDI. It appears to be the most effective treatment for prevention of recurrent infection, so it stands to reason that it should be similarly effective for treatment of primary infection or prevention of a first recurrence. In many cases, diarrhea caused by *C. difficile* is characterized by debilitating symptoms that include extreme fecal urgency and episodes of fecal incontinence, abdominal cramps, high frequency of bowel movements during the day and night, and exhaustion. Patients often become terrified that the infection may return, knowing that there is a 20% to 30% chance of recurrence following initial treatment of CDI.[2] Several perspectives need to be considered in answering this question: scientific, financial, and legal. This section outlines the role of FMT for primary CDI.

It is important to emphasize that at this time, FMT is generally offered following antibiotic treatment, typically vancomycin, and used to prevent further CDI recurrence. It is assumed that success of FMT is at least partially dependent on prior antibiotic-mediated suppression of vegetative *C. difficile* bacteria-producing toxins, while FMT restores the

Allegretti JR, Kassam Z, eds. *The 6 Ds of Fecal Microbiota Transplantation: A Primer From Decision to Discharge and Beyond* (pp 105-110). © 2021 SLACK Incorporated.

intestinal microbial community structure and microbiota-mediated colonization resistance to *C. difficile*.[3] Recently, a small proof-of-concept trial compared metronidazole treatment with FMT delivered via enema (60 mL, anaerobically prepared) for the treatment of primary CDI (Figure 10.1.1-1).[4] The primary outcome was clinical cure, defined as < 3 bowel movements per day and no evidence of recurrence at day 70. Overall, 5 of 9 patients responded to treatment in the FMT arm, which was comparable to 5 of 11 responders in the metronidazole group. By day 4 after treatment, the remaining 4 FMT patients were given metronidazole, only 2 of whom had adequate secondary response. From a safety perspective, there were no safety events in either arm. There were some limitations with this study, beyond the small sample size. Specifically, the investigators compared metronidazole with FMT administered by enema. Notably, metronidazole is no longer recommended for primary therapy of CDI in adults because of lesser efficacy and greater side effects compared with other antibiotics.[3] In addition, administration of FMT by enema may be less efficacious relative to other routes, such as colonoscopy or capsule.[5] The investigators are now conducting a Phase 3 trial to evaluate FMT as a primary treatment of CDI.

Importantly, fulminant CDI, which commonly presents as primary infection, must be regarded as a distinct clinical entity. It is a disease characterized by high mortality and morbidity and needs to be treated in the most urgent manner. FMT is an important consideration in management of this CDI presentation, and this topic is covered in much greater detail in Chapter 10.1.2: "The Role of Fecal Microbiota Transplantation in the Treatment of Severe and Fulminant *Clostridioides difficile* Infection." Briefly, in our unique University of Minnesota experience, in a series of 16 patients (unpublished), some of the most common factors that are associated with poor outcomes in fulminant CDI management include late recognition of disease severity and delayed specialist consultation, concurrent use of broad-spectrum antibiotics for sepsis (typically without another source), and use of narcotics for pain control. In our center, we offer FMT after failure to document clinical benefit following at least 48 hours of appropriate medical therapy. In most cases, FMT leads to prompt improvement within 24 to 48 hours of FMT by colonoscopy, which is documented by clinical signs and symptoms, hemodynamic parameters, and inflammatory markers. Importantly, FMT in treatment of fulminant CDI generally needs to be administered more than once because of high risk of recurrence following a single treatment.[6,7] Our current FMT protocol for fulminant CDI includes (1) specialist consensus (gastroenterology, infectious disease, and colorectal surgery); (2) discontinuation of all antibiotics;

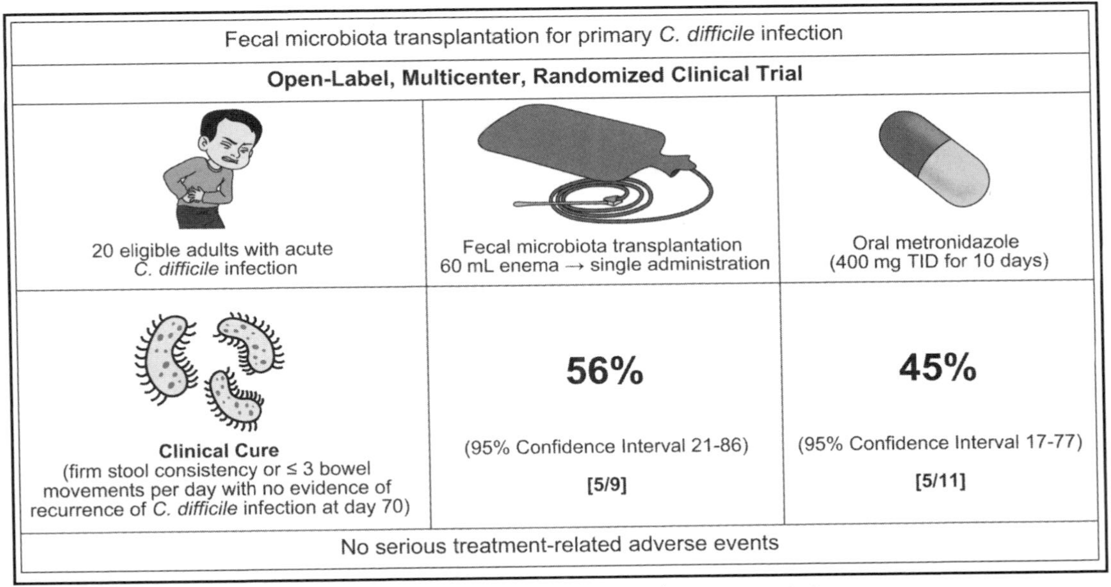

Figure 10.1.1-1. Fecal microbiota transplantation for primary *C. difficile* infection.[4] (TID = 3 times/day.)

Fecal microbiota transplantation for primary *C. difficile* infection

Open-Label, Multicenter, Randomized Clinical Trial

20 eligible adults with acute *C. difficile* infection	Fecal microbiota transplantation 60 mL enema → single administration	Oral metronidazole (400 mg TID for 10 days)
Clinical Cure (firm stool consistency or ≤ 3 bowel movements per day with no evidence of recurrence of *C. difficile* infection at day 70)	**56%** (95% Confidence Interval 21-86) [5/9]	**45%** (95% Confidence Interval 17-77) [5/11]
No serious treatment-related adverse events		

followed by (3) FMT by colonoscopy as initial treatment; (4) resumption of antibiotics against CDI (vancomycin or fidaxomicin) 3 days after the initial FMT (patients are typically discharged from the hospital shortly after); and finally (5) a consolidation treatment with FMT by capsules given on an outpatient basis. The initial colonoscopic delivery of FMT is important for documentation of pseudomembranous colitis, because it is not uncommon to see fulminant CDI-like clinical presentation where the septic picture is driven by another source. The goal of this initial treatment is clinical stabilization. Once the patient is discharged, the syndrome can be considered equivalent to outpatient rCDI, where the remaining treatment goal is prevention of CDI recurrence. Logistically, oral capsules provide the easiest formulation for most such patients.

Recently, we evaluated the cost-effectiveness of different treatments for CDI and rCDI within the context of the latest guidelines from the Infectious Diseases Society of America (IDSA).[8,9] These guidelines include a variety of treatment options and take into consideration some clinical factors, such as disease severity and history of recurrence. Cost-effectiveness is not a primary consideration in clinical guidelines, but cost remains a critical factor in many health care settings. Our modeling was based on medication costs, including cost of FMT as provided by the Centers for Medicare & Medicaid Services, as well as that reported in previous studies and hospitalization costs. We found fidaxomicin to be the most effective strategy for primary, non-severe CDI; vancomycin for primary, severe CDI; fidaxomicin for first recurrence of CDI; and FMT for subsequent recurrence. Modeling permutations showed that FMT was no longer cost-effective when priced at $\geq \$14,800$.[9] Of course, pure cost calculations do not translate into preferred clinical algorithms in practice, which may explain poor market penetration by fidaxomicin in treatment of CDI. Payers continue to require prior failure of vancomycin, and high copays discourage its use even when those therapies have failed. Although not examined in this study, the use of FMT in primary CDI may potentially be beneficial in high-risk groups, such as those with underlying IBD.

The legal issue is arguably the most straightforward. Under the current enforcement discretion policy, still in force at the time of this writing, the US Food and Drug Administration (FDA) allows use of FMT in treatment of CDI that does not respond to standard therapies (ie, antibiotics), without regulatory requirements that are generally mandatory for investigational drugs. The latest guidelines from the IDSA recommend FMT after the second or subsequent recurrence of CDI.[8]

Practical Pearl 10.1.1-1

Microbiome Therapeutics

- A major deficiency in most FMT studies thus far has been a paucity of evaluation of pharmacokinetic (PK) and pharmacodynamic (PD) parameters.
- The focus has been mainly on clinical outcomes, which are critically important. However, absence of PK/PD studies makes it difficult to compare FMT and other microbiome therapeutic products, determine the ideal dose/dose regimen, and continue to progress in the field.
- PK studies of microbiome therapeutics should include quantitative assessment of donor bacteria engraftment, as measured in fecal samples collected over time.
- PD studies will vary by disease indication but should evaluate changes in the overall intestinal microbial community structure and an evaluation of key disease-specific biomarkers.

Looking toward the future, we should recognize that the modern history of microbiome therapeutics, including FMT, started only within the past decade. FMT and microbiome therapeutics may be a therapeutic option for primary CDI; however, further research is required, and ongoing clinical trials are needed (Practical Pearl 10.1.1-1).

Summary

The role of FMT in primary CDI is still under investigation; however, pilot data suggests this may be a promising approach. Patients with primary CDI that are in a high-risk group, such as those with comorbid IBD, who are at an increased risk of poor outcomes, may benefit the most from novel therapeutics. Larger trials that are adequately controlled are needed to further explore the use of FMT in primary CDI.

References

1. Oren A, Rupnik M. *Clostridium difficile* and *Clostridioides difficile*: two validly published and correct names. *Anaerobe.* 2018;52:125-126.
2. Louie TJ, Miller MA, Mullane KM, et al. Fidaxomicin versus vancomycin for *Clostridium difficile* infection. *N Engl J Med.* 2011;364(5):422-431.

3. Khoruts A, Sadowsky MJ. Understanding the mechanisms of faecal microbiota transplantation. *Nat Rev Gastroenterol Hepatol.* 2016;13(9):508-516.

4. Juul FE, Garborg K, Bretthauer M, et al. Fecal microbiota transplantation for primary *Clostridium difficile* infection. *N Engl J Med.* 2018;378(26):2535-2536.

5. Tariq R, Pardi DS, Bartlett MG, Khanna S. Low cure rates in controlled trials of fecal microbiota transplantation for recurrent *Clostridium difficile* infection: a systematic review and meta-analysis. *Clin Infect Dis.* 2019;68(8):1351-1358.

6. Weingarden AR, Hamilton MJ, Sadowsky MJ, Khoruts A. Resolution of severe *Clostridium difficile* infection following sequential fecal microbiota transplantation. *J Clin Gastroenterol.* 2013;47(8):735-737.

7. Fischer M, Sipe B, Cheng YW, et al. Fecal microbiota transplant in severe and severe-complicated *Clostridium difficile*: a promising treatment approach. *Gut Microbes.* 2016;8(3):289-302.

8. McDonald LC, Gerding DN, Johnson S, et al. Clinical practice guidelines for *Clostridium difficile* infection in adults and children: 2017 update by the Infectious Diseases Society of America (IDSA) and Society for Healthcare Epidemiology of America (SHEA). *Clin Infect Dis.* 2018;66(7):987-994.

9. Rajasingham R, Enns EA, Khoruts A, Vaughn BP. Cost-effectiveness of treatment regimens for *Clostridioides difficile* infection—an evaluation of the 2018 Infectious Diseases Society of America guidelines. *Clin Infect Dis.* 2020;70(5):754-762.

10.1

10.1.2 The Role of Fecal Microbiota Transplantation in the Treatment of Severe and Fulminant *Clostridioides difficile* Infection

Monika Fischer, MD, MSc and Sára Nemes, BA

    Clostridioides difficile infection (CDI; previously *Clostridium difficile* infection) is the leading cause of nosocomial infections, and its associated morbidity and mortality have dramatically increased since 2000.[1] Identification and implementation of effective treatment modalities is imperative, particularly in patients with severe or fulminant CDI, to decrease the need for surgical intervention and reduce high mortality rates, length of intensive care unit (ICU) and hospital stays, and hospital readmission rates.[2] In several case series, cohort studies, and randomized trials, FMT has emerged as a promising therapy for the treatment of severe and fulminant CDI, with cure rates as high as 70% to 90% with repeated administration and/or concomitant antibiotics.[2-6] In this section, we outline the role of FMT in severe and fulminant CDI.

Defining Severe and Fulminant *Clostridioides difficile* Infection

    In approximately 8% to 12% of cases, CDI presents as a state of life-threatening systemic toxicity.[7] These severe and fulminant cases

Allegretti JR, Kassam Z, eds. *The 6 Ds of Fecal Microbiota Transplantation: A Primer From Decision to Discharge and Beyond* (pp 111-117).

Table 10.1.2-1. Definition of Severe and Fulminant *Clostridioides difficile* Infection: Infectious Diseases Society of America and American College of Gastroenterology Guidelines

Severity	IDSA/SHEA (2018)	ACG (2013)
Severe	• White blood cells ≥ 15,000/μl *or* creatinine ≥ 1.5	• Serum albumin < 3 g/dL *plus* ≥ 1 of the following: ° White blood cells ≥ 15,000/μL ° Abdominal tenderness
Fulminant	• Hypotension or shock • Ileus • Megacolon	• ≥ 1 attributable to CDI • ICU admission • Hypotension • Fever ≥ 38.5° C • Ileus • Mental status changes • White blood cells ≥ 35,000/μL or < 2,000/μL • Serum lactate > 2.2 mmol/L • End organ failure

Abbreviations: ACG = American College of Gastroenterology; SHEA = Society for Healthcare Epidemiology of America.

Adapted from McDonald et al[1] and Surawicz et al.[9]

of CDI may result in ICU admission, sepsis, toxic megacolon, significant organ dysfunction, and death.[8] Although there is not a unified consensus on the definition of severe and fulminant CDI, several medical society guidelines provide clarity on how to define these patients (Table 10.1.2-1).

Identifying patients who are at risk of developing severe or fulminant CDI early in the disease course may mitigate poor outcomes. Clinical scores, such as the *C. difficile*–Associated Risk of Death Score, can be used to predict risk of death in CDI.[10,11] In a large retrospective review of 336 patients, Henrich et al[11] identified several risk factors associated with development of severe CDI, including age over 70 years (odds ratio [OR], 3.35), maximum leukocyte count over 20,000 cells/mL (OR, 2.77), minimum serum albumin less than 2.5 g/dL (OR, 3.44), maximum serum creatinine over 2 mg/dL (OR, 2.47), small bowel obstruction or ileus (OR,

3.06), and colorectal inflammation on computed tomography imaging (OR, 13.54). Additional risk factors for poor outcomes include the presence of the epidemic NAP/027/BI strain,[12,13] possibly high fecal *C. difficile* toxin levels,[14] and a lower median cycle threshold during nucleic acid amplification testing of the stool sample.[15]

Surgical Intervention for *Clostridioides difficile* Infection

Current mainstream therapy for patients with severe or fulminant CDI refractory to maximum medical therapy (oral vancomycin 500 mg 4 times/day, intravenous metronidazole 500 mg 3/day, and vancomycin enemas in case of ileus) is surgery. Without surgery, the in-hospital mortality rate of these cases approaches 80% to 90%.[16] Up to 30% of severe and fulminant CDI eventually may require colectomy.[17] Outcomes following colectomy are poor, with 30-day mortality rates as high 35% to 57%.[18,19] Moreover, many patients who develop severe or fulminant CDI are not ideal candidates for surgical intervention due to underlying comorbidities that predict poor post-surgical outcomes, including acute respiratory failure, renal failure, thrombocytopenia, and chronic obstructive pulmonary disease.[20] Suboptimal surgical candidates may qualify for less invasive loop ileostomy followed by anterograde vancomycin lavage. In 2011, a randomized clinical trial showed a 31% reduction in 30-day perioperative mortality when loop ileostomy was performed, with preservation of the colon in 93% of patients.[7] From 2011 to 2015, the annual proportion of loop ileostomy performed for fulminant CDI increased from 11% to 25% in US hospitals, with no difference in in-hospital mortality or length of stay compared with those undergoing total abdominal colectomy.[21] Surgical-site disruption and operative wound were also more common in the patients with loop ileostomy. Selection bias (deciding for loop ileostomy in sicker patients), at least in part, may be responsible for these outcomes.

Fecal Microbiota Transplantation as Treatment for Severe and Fulminant *Clostridioides difficile* Infection

A pseudomembrane-driven protocol published by Fischer et al[22] (Figure 10.1.2-1) emphasizes the need for sequential FMTs and selective use of oral vancomycin. As described in this protocol, patients receive oral vancomycin for a minimum of 48 hours (in clinical practice for

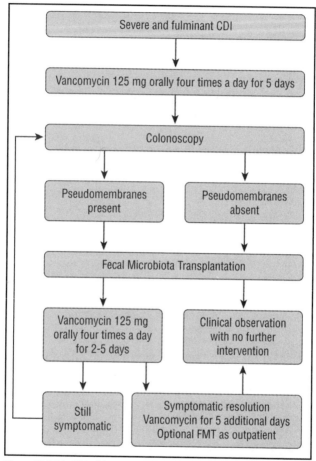

Figure 10.1.2-1. Clinical framework for management of severe and fulminant *C. difficile* infection patients with fecal microbiota transplantation. (Adapted from Fischer et al.[2])

an average of 5 days) before undergoing an FMT by colonoscopy by a skilled endoscopist. If pseudomembranes are identified, oral vancomycin is to be restarted 48 hours following FMT. In the presence of continued CDI symptoms 3 to 5 days following the procedure, the FMT is to be repeated. This sequence of procedures should continue in the described 3- to 5-day intervals until pseudomembranes resolve.[22] Among the 57 patients who underwent this protocol, only 12% required 3 or more FMTs, according to a retrospective analysis. Promisingly, the clinical cure rate was 100% for severe CDI and 87% for fulminant CDI, and no related serious adverse events were reported.[2] These data suggest that clinical rates of treating severe and fulminant CDI may be similar to that of non-severe rCDI as long as antibiotics and successive FMTs are appropriately used. The need for multiple FMTs is likely due to the higher *C. difficile* burden present in severe CDI. Although a single FMT is often insufficient to achieve complete clinical cure, in theory it restores the microbial scaffolding enabling antibiotics to be more successful. Vancomycin is the most commonly used antibiotic in this clinical setting; however, fidaxomicin may also be used, given that it has a more narrow spectrum.

Ianiro et al[23] applied a similar protocol in an open-label randomized clinical trial. In their protocol, a single FMT in combination with a 14-day course of vancomycin was compared with multiple FMTs repeated every 3 days in combination with a 14-day course of vancomycin. The overall clinical cure rate was 75% (21/28) for the single FMT group and 100% (28/28) for the multiple FMT group (*P* = .01), the latter group containing 57% fulminant CDI cases. No serious related adverse events were noted in either study.

Although FMT can be administered through alternative routes, colonoscopy is the preferred mode of administration for severe and fulminant CDI. Given the risk of potentially fatal ileus-associated aspiration, FMT administration by upper GI route, including capsules, in critically ill patients is not advised.[2] Enemas are often insufficient and are not retained for the desired length of time due to poor rectal sphincter tone. Additionally, enemas do not allow for assessment of the mucosal response. The presence of stool banks have streamlined the process of administering FMTs, making the treatment available and increasing the safety profile through extensive donor and stool testing.[24]

FMT may be particularly beneficial for patients who are considered unfit for surgery. This category of patients should receive FMT as salvage therapy. In critically ill, unstable patients, FMT may help to stabilize them prior to colectomy if surgery is considered to be the treatment of choice. In this situation, FMT should be considered as adjunctive therapy to successful surgery. FMT may be easily administered in the ICU without delaying colectomy.[25]

There are limitations of FMT as a treatment in this patient cohort. Among severe and fulminant patients, 2 phenotypes have emerged as not being candidates for FMT: patients experiencing multiorgan failure refractory to supportive therapy and acidosis (pH <7.2) and those with toxic megacolon and signs of impending perforation.[26] Careful consideration and evidence-guided decision making is essential in identifying patients who would not benefit from FMT.

Summary

FMT optimizes the treatment of severe and fulminant CDI by decreasing mortality rates and need for colectomy. In conjunction with antibiotics, application of sequential FMT protocol in patients with pseudomembranous colitis may increase cure rate to 70% to 90%. Validation of these data in randomized placebo-controlled trials would be ideal, but execution of such trials proves to be challenging in the critically ill patient population.

References

1. McDonald LC, Gerding DN, Johnson S, et al. Clinical practice guidelines for *Clostridium difficile* infection in adults and children: 2017 update by the Infectious Diseases Society of America (IDSA) and Society for Healthcare Epidemiology of America (SHEA). *Clin Infect Dis*. 2018;66(7):e1-e48.

2. Fischer M, Sipe B, Cheng YW, et al. Fecal microbiota transplant in severe and severe-complicated *Clostridium difficile*: a promising treatment approach. *Gut Microbes*. 2017;8(3):289-302.

3. Ianiro G, Maida M, Burisch J, et al. Efficacy of different faecal microbiota transplantation protocols for *Clostridium difficile* infection: a systematic review and meta-analysis. *United European Gastroenterol J*. 2018;6(8):1232-1244.

4. Cammarota G, Masucci L, Ianiro G, et al. Randomised clinical trial: faecal microbiota transplantation by colonoscopy vs. vancomycin for the treatment of recurrent *Clostridium difficile* infection. *Aliment Pharmacol Ther*. 2015;41(9):835-843.

5. Cammarota G, Ianiro G, Magalini S, Gasbarrini A, Gui D. Decrease in surgery for *Clostridium difficile* infection after starting a program to transplant fecal microbiota. *Ann Intern Med*. 2015;163(6):487-488.

6. Agrawal M, Aroniadis OC, Brandt LJ, et al. The long-term efficacy and safety of fecal microbiota transplant for recurrent, severe, and complicated *Clostridium difficile* infection in 146 elderly individuals. *J Clin Gastroenterol*. 2016;50(5):403-407.

7. Neal MD, Alverdy JC, Hall DE, Simmons RL, Zuckerbraun BS. Diverting loop ileostomy and colonic lavage: an alternative to total abdominal colectomy for the treatment of severe, complicated *Clostridium difficile* associated disease. *Ann Surg*. 2011;254(3):423-429.

8. Dallal RM, Harbrecht BG, Boujoukas AJ, et al. Fulminant *Clostridium difficile*: an underappreciated and increasing cause of death and complications. *Ann Surg*. 2002;235(3):363-372.

9. Surawicz CM, Brandt LJ, Binion DG, et al. Guidelines for diagnosis, treatment, and prevention of Clostridium difficile infections. *Am J Gastroenterol.* 2013;108:478-98.

10. Kassam Z, Cribb Fabersunne C, Smith MB, et al. *Clostridium difficile* Associated Risk of Death Score (CARDS): a novel severity score to predict mortality among hospitalised patients with *C. difficile* infection. *Aliment Pharmacol Ther.* 2016;43(6):725-733.

11. Henrich TJ, Krakower D, Bitton A, Yokoe DS. Clinical risk factors for severe *Clostridium difficile*-associated disease. *Emerg Infect Dis.* 2009;15(3):415-422.

12. See I, Mu Y, Cohen J, et al. NAP1 strain type predicts outcomes from *Clostridium difficile* infection. *Clin Infect Dis.* 2014;58(10):1394-1400.

13. Miller M, Gravel D, Mulvey M, et al. Health care-associated *Clostridium difficile* infection in Canada: patient age and infecting strain type are highly predictive of severe outcome and mortality. *Clin Infect Dis.* 2010;50(2):194-201.

14. Cohen NA, Miller T, Na'aminh W, et al. *Clostridium difficile* fecal toxin level is associated with disease severity and prognosis. *United European Gastroenterol J.* 2018;6(5):773-780.

15. Davies KA, Planche T, Wilcox MH. The predictive value of quantitative nucleic acid amplification detection of *Clostridium difficile* toxin gene for faecal sample toxin status and patient outcome. *PLoS One.* 2018;13(12):e0205941.

16. Bhangu S, Bhangu A, Nightingale P, Michael A. Mortality and risk stratification in patients with *Clostridium difficile*-associated diarrhoea. *Colorectal Dis.* 2010;12(3):241-246.

17. Bhangu A, Nepogodiev D, Gupta A, Torrance A, Singh P; West Midlands Research Collaborative. Systematic review and meta-analysis of outcomes following emergency surgery for *Clostridium difficile* colitis. *Br J Surg.* 2012;99(11):1501-1513.

18. Seder CW, Villalba MR Jr, Robbins J, et al. Early colectomy may be associated with improved survival in fulminant *Clostridium difficile* colitis: an 8-year experience. *Am J Surg.* 2009;197(3):302-307.

19. Stewart DB, Hollenbeak CS, Wilson MZ. Is colectomy for fulminant *Clostridium difficile* colitis life saving? A systematic review. *Colorectal Dis.* 2013;15(7):798-804.

20. Hall JF, Berger D. Outcome of colectomy for *Clostridium difficile* colitis: a plea for early surgical management. *Am J Surg.* 2008;196(3):384-388.

21. Juo YY, Sanaiha Y, Jabaji Z, Benharash P. Trends in diverting loop ileostomy vs total abdominal colectomy as surgical management for *Clostridium difficile* colitis. *JAMA Surg.* 2019;154(10):899-906.

22. Fischer M, Sipe BW, Rogers NA, et al. Faecal microbiota transplantation plus selected use of vancomycin for severe-complicated *Clostridium difficile* infection: description of a protocol with high success rate. *Aliment Pharmacol Ther.* 2015;42(4):470-476.

23. Ianiro G, Masucci L, Quaranta G, et al. Randomised clinical trial: faecal microbiota transplantation by colonoscopy plus vancomycin for the treatment of severe refractory *Clostridium difficile* infection—single versus multiple infusions. *Aliment Pharmacol Ther.* 2018;48(2):152-159.

24. Kassam Z, Dubois N, Ramakrishna B, et al. Donor screening for fecal microbiota transplantation. *N Engl J Med.* 2019;381(21):2070-2072.

25. Clanton J, Fawley R, Haller N, et al. Patience is a virtue: an argument for delayed surgical intervention in fulminant *Clostridium difficile* colitis. *Am Surg.* 2014;80(6):614-619.

26. Fischer M, Kao D, Mehta SR, et al. Predictors of early failure after fecal microbiota transplantation for the therapy of *Clostridium difficile* infection: a multicenter study. *Am J Gastroenterol.* 2016;111(7):1024-1031.

10.2

Gastrointestinal Indications
What Have We Learned?

10.2.1 The Role of Fecal Microbiota Transplantation in the Treatment of Inflammatory Bowel Disease

*Lindsey Russell, MD, MSc and
Paul Moayyedi, MD, PhD, MPH*

IBD is thought to arise from a dysregulated immune system reacting to an environmental agent in a genetically susceptible individual. Most therapies currently focus on dampening the immune response, with very little attention paid to possible environmental stimulus driving the inflammation that characterizes IBD.[1] Our ability to study the microbiome has increased exponentially over the past decade, and this has allowed us to understand differences in the microbiome in patients with IBD compared with those who are healthy.[2] Indeed, it is likely that the microbiome is driving the immune response in IBD, and if the gut microbiota were altered in a favorable direction, this could ameliorate the disease. Researchers have attempted to do this with antibiotics[3] and probiotics but with limited success. This is not surprising because we have a limited understanding of what constitutes a healthy microbiome so cannot engineer this with antibiotics or probiotics.

Altering the gut microbiota in IBD patients with microbiota from a healthy donor by FMT is an intuitive approach to this problem. Even if we cannot define a healthy gut microbiota, we may able to restore homeostasis through FMT and thus treat IBD patients. This section will review the

Allegretti JR, Kassam Z, eds. *The 6 Ds of Fecal Microbiota Transplantation: A Primer From Decision to Discharge and Beyond* (pp 118-123).
© 2021 SLACK Incorporated.

evidence for FMT in the 2 diseases that constitute IBD—ulcerative colitis (UC) and Crohn's disease (CD)—as well as give future directions for study.

Fecal Microbiota Transplantation in Ulcerative Colitis

There is more evidence for the efficacy of FMT in UC than any other disease except CDI. There are 4 randomized clinical trials that have evaluated FMT in 277 active UC patients,[4-7] and 3 trials have been positive.[5-7] A systematic review suggested that FMT induces remission in approximately 25% of patients with active UC compared with 5% of those given placebo after 6 to 8 weeks.[8] This translates to a number needed to treat (NNT) of 5 (95% confidence interval,[4-10]; Figure 10.2.1-1), which is similar to the NNT seen for biologic therapy.[9] The evidence has been assessed according to Grading of Recommendations, Assessment, Development and Evaluations criteria[9] and is low-quality evidence because there is imprecision in the estimate and there is heterogeneity between studies in terms of type of donor, mode of administration, and type of active UC patient included in the trial. Interestingly, 1 trial suggested there may be a donor effect, with 1 donor being effective in 40% of cases while another donor was not successful in any patient.[5] This trial also suggested that FMT may be more effective in those who had been diagnosed with UC within 1 year and those who were taking concomitant immunosuppressive therapy but had flared despite taking these drugs.[5] These observations are based on small numbers of patients and need evaluation in further trials. The longest follow-up for FMT in the context of a randomized trial was 1 year; therefore, further follow-up is needed to establish the long-term benefit of this approach. In our experience, most patients flare over time but usually respond to further courses of FMT. Currently, we offer UC patients who are in remission with FMT repeated enemas every 2 to 4 weeks as maintenance therapy, although this is still investigational (Figure 10.2.1-2).

Fecal Microbiota Transplantation in Crohn's Disease

There is less evidence for the role of FMT in CD than there is for UC. There is only 1 randomized clinical trial, and it compared administering FMT via gastroscopy or colonoscopy with no placebo arm.[10] One study found that FMT increased microbial diversity in CD patients, and this was more apparent in patients who responded to therapy.[11] A systematic review of case series of active CD patients treated with FMT identified 11 studies that reported that 52% (95% confidence interval, 31%-72%)

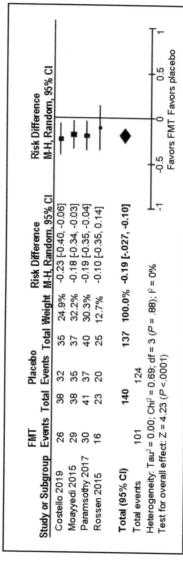

Figure 10.2.1-1. Forest plot of efficacy of fecal microbiota transplantation in inducing remission in active ulcerative colitis.[4-7]

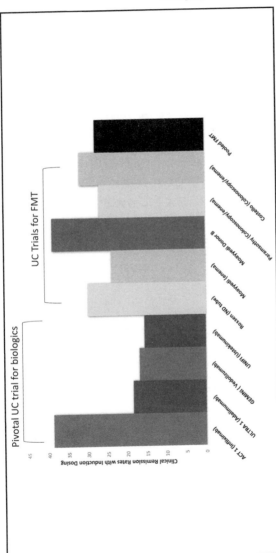

Figure 10.2.1-2. Clinical remission rates from randomized clinical trials assessing biologic therapy or fecal microbiota transplantation for the induction of remission of ulcerative colitis. Note: Eligibility and definition of clinical remission vary by study.[4-7,15,16] (ND=nasoduodenal.)

achieved clinical remission.[12] There was significant clinical and statistical heterogeneity between studies, and most studies did not perform a colonoscopy at the end of treatment, so the impact on mucosal healing is less certain. The choice of donor and mode of delivery was also different between studies, with some using colonoscopy, others using nasogastric tubes (NGTs), and yet others using capsules to deliver FMT. Open-label studies where there is no control arm almost always overestimate treatment effect, so it is unclear whether FMT is effective in active CD. Case series data are promising, and there are a number of randomized trials of FMT in active CD currently being conducted.

Future Directions for Fecal Microbiota Transplantation in Inflammatory Bowel Disease

Currently there is insufficient evidence for FMT to be used in clinical practice to treat IBD, and more evidence is needed. Unlike in the prevention of CDI, 1 dose is not sufficient to treat IBD, but the optimum frequency and duration is unclear. It appears that once-weekly FMT is as effective as more frequent administration,[5,6] but the length of time needed to treat before maximizing response has not been determined. The ideal mode of delivery needs to be established and whether lyophilized, fresh, or frozen stool is equally effective. Lyophilized FMT material is as effective as frozen for CDI,[13] and if this is also true for IBD, this will make FMT easier to administer in the hospital setting and make it more feasible for patients to use at home and while traveling. FMT via retention enema may also be sufficient for UC. Utilization of noncolonoscopic administration will be important because it is likely that IBD will require more than 1 dose. CD will probably need to be administered by FMT capsules if regular dosing is needed, because neither colonoscopic nor endoscopic administration is feasible for repeated doses. Finally, there is the issue of donor specificity. Unlike CDI, response may be donor specific, and future studies should evaluate the microbiome of donors and recipients in detail to determine what is driving the success of this approach. This may lead to more targeted, curated organisms used in IBD, and there are pilot randomized clinical trial data to suggest this may be effective and may be enhanced by adding vancomycin for 6 days before giving the first FMT treatment.[14]

Summary

The evidence is not of sufficient quality to recommend FMT for either UC or CD outside of a clinical study at this time. Initial data are promising, and microbiome therapeutics such as FMT may become a treatment option if research can optimize how this should be used and if larger trials allow us to be more confident that it can induce remission in patients with active disease. There is an increasing amount of research in FMT in IBD, and the future looks bright for this being an option for patients.

References

1. Moayyedi P. Fecal transplantation: any real hope for inflammatory bowel disease? *Curr Opin Gastroenterol*. 2016;32(4):282-286.

2. Pittayanon R, Lau JT, Leontiadis GI, et al. Differences in gut microbiota in patients with vs without inflammatory bowel diseases: a systematic review. *Gastroenterology*. 2020;158(4):930-946.e1.

3. Khan KJ, Ullman TA, Ford AC, et al. Antibiotic therapy in inflammatory bowel disease: a systematic review and meta-analysis. *Am J Gastroenterol*. 2011;106(4):661-673.

4. Rossen NG, Fuentes S, van der Spek MJ, et al. Findings from a randomized controlled trial of fecal transplantation for patients with ulcerative colitis. *Gastroenterology*. 2015;149(1):110-118.e4.

5. Moayyedi P, Surette MG, Kim PT, et al. Fecal microbiota transplantation induces remission in patients with active ulcerative colitis in a randomized controlled trial. *Gastroenterology*. 2015;149(1):102-109.e6.

6. Paramsothy S, Kamm MA, Kaakoush NO, et al. Multidonor intensive faecal microbiota transplantation for active ulcerative colitis: a randomised placebo-controlled trial. *Lancet*. 2017;389(10075):1218-1228.

7. Costello SP, Hughes P, Waters O, et al. Effect of fecal microbiota transplantation on 8-week remission in patients with ulcerative colitis: a randomized clinical trial. *JAMA*. 2019;321(2):156-164.

8. Narula N, Kassam Z, Yuan YH, et al. Systematic review and meta-analysis: fecal microbiota transplantation for treatment of active ulcerative colitis. *Inflamm Bowel Dis*. 2017;23(10):1702-1709.

9. Talley NJ, Abreu MT, Achkar JP, et al. An evidence-based systematic review on medical therapies in inflammatory bowel disease. *Am J Gastroenterol*. 2011;106 (suppl 1):S2-S26.

10. Yang Z, Bu C, Yuan W, et al. Fecal microbiota transplant via endoscopic delivering through small intestine and colon: no difference for Crohn's disease. *Dig Dis Sci*. 2020;65(1):150-157.

11. Vaughn BP, Vatanen T, Allegretti JR, et al. Increased intestinal microbial diversity following fecal microbiota transplant for active Crohn's disease. *Inflamm Bowel Dis*. 2016;22(9):2182-2190.

12. Paramsothy S, Paramsothy R, Rubin DT, et al. Faecal microbiota transplantation for inflammatory bowel disease: a systematic review and meta-analysis. *J Crohns Colitis*. 2017;11(10):1180-1199.

13. Lee CH, Steiner T, Petrof EO, et al. Frozen vs fresh fecal microbiota transplantation and clinical resolution of diarrhea in patients with recurrent *Clostridium difficile* infection: a randomized clinical trial. *JAMA*. 2016;315(2):142-149.

14. Misra B, Curran J, Herfarth H, et al. P421 SER-287, an investigational microbiome therapeutic, induces remission and endoscopic improvement in a placebo-controlled, double-blind randomised trial in patients with active mild-to-moderate ulcerative colitis. *J Crohns Colitis*. 2018;12(suppl 1):S317.

15. Rutgeerts P, Sandborn WJ, Feagan BG, et al. Infliximab for induction and maintenance therapy for ulcerative colitis. *N Engl J Med*. 2005;353:2462-2476.

16. Reinisch W, Sandborn WJ, Hommes DW, et al. Adalimumab for induction of clinical remission in moderately to severely active ulcerative colitis: results of a randomized controlled trial. *Gut*. 2011;60:780-787.

10.2

10.2.2 The Role of Fecal Microbiota Transplantation in the Treatment of Pouchitis

Jennifer D. Claytor, MD, MS and Najwa El-Nachef, MD

Pouchitis is a common complication after ileal pouch–anal anastomosis (IPAA) surgery for UC, occurring in up to 40% to 50% of patients (Figure 10.2.2-1)[1]; 10% to 20% of these patients develop chronic symptoms requiring prolonged antibiotic.[1,2] Although the pathogenesis of pouchitis is not well understood, it is hypothesized that the intestinal microbiome plays a key role. This is supported by the role of antibiotics in the successful treatment of pouchitis, as well as the role of probiotics in preventing pouchitis recurrence.

FMT is being explored as a promising new therapy for IBD, with preliminary favorable safety and therapeutic profiles for UC.[3] Given that the microbial milieu of the pouch is more colon-like than ileal,[4] a similar response to FMT in pouchitis and UC is hypothesized. However, much remains to be clarified, including the optimal dosing route and frequency of FMT; appropriate patient and donor selection; and markers, such as donor stool microbiota engraftment, that may predict clinical and endoscopic response. In this section, we outline the role of FMT for pouchitis.

Allegretti JR, Kassam Z, eds. *The 6 Ds of Fecal Microbiota Transplantation: A Primer From Decision to Discharge and Beyond* (pp 124-131).
© 2021 SLACK Incorporated.

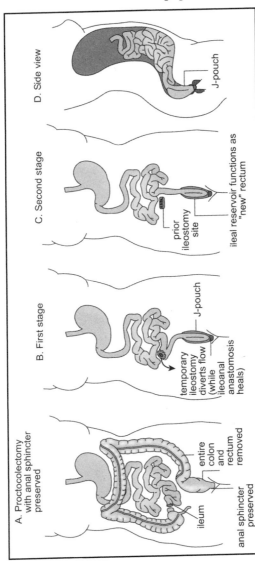

Figure 10.2.2-1. Construction of an ileoanal pouch anastomosis.

Patient Selection

To date, all case reports and prospective studies have been limited by small numbers of participants, with 55 total reported in clinical FMT studies (Table 10.2.2-1).[4-11] Heterogeneity in inclusion criteria limits comparison across studies, and the studies vary in baseline Pouchitis Disease Activity Index (PDAI) scores. In a small case series, patients with a high baseline PDAI had the most promising clinical outcomes. Selvig et al[10] presented data on 19 patients with a baseline mean PDAI of 7. The authors reported that patients had a statistically significant improvement in bowel movements and abdominal pain. There was no significant change in endoscopic or histologic outcomes; however, these results are difficult to assess given some patients were in clinical remission at baseline.[10] Interestingly, they noted that patients did have a statistically significant improvement in bowel movements and abdominal pain, which may have resulted from addressing irritable pouch syndrome.

Future studies should investigate whether the microbial milieu of patients with more severe pouchitis is more amenable to FMT than those with quiescent disease. If so, this would differ from patients with severe UC, who may be less likely to achieve endoscopic or clinical benefit from FMT.[12] In patients with mild pouchitis at the onset, it is possible that their symptoms may be due to bacterial overgrowth or irritable pouch syndrome, and data suggest that FMT may be beneficial in patients with IBS (see Chapter 10.2.3: "The Role of Fecal Microbiota Transplantation in the Treatment of Irritable Bowel Syndrome").

Donor Selection

Major questions remain regarding optimal donor selection, including preparation, impact of pooled vs individual donors, and fresh vs frozen material (see Table 10.2.2-1). Interestingly, Stallmach et al[6] reported that a pouchitis patient eventually achieved remission, but only after switching the FMT donor. These results support the donor specific effect observed by Moayyedi et al,[13] who noted that 1 donor (Donor B) induced remission in patients with active UC compared with any other donor.

Two recent studies used frozen FMT material, with Selvig et al[10] reporting no donor specific effect among 13 individual donors. Herfarth et al[9] selected a single donor based on a high concentration of butyrate-producing bacteria. Butyrate has previously been shown to have an anti-inflammatory effect in UC.[14] However, despite selecting for butyrate enrichment, the study was terminated due to lack of benefit. Landy et al[5] noted increased butyrate on 1H nuclear magnetic resonance spectroscopy but similarly failed to induction clinical or endoscopic remission.

Mode and Timing of Fecal Microbiota Transplantation Delivery

Uncertainty remains regarding the optimal protocol for delivery of FMT to target pouchitis. FMT by pouchoscopy every 3 weeks produced the greatest clinical benefit, with 80% remission after the third dose.[7] One study investigated a bowel lavage and 5-day course of rifaximin prior to FMT by pouchoscopy, aiming to enhance engraftment; although fewer bowel movements and less abdominal pain were noted, there was no significant improvement in histologic or endoscopic scores.[10] Oral FMT capsules have great potential as a feasible and patient-friendly means of maintaining remission, if individual donor and recipient factors can be optimized. In a pilot study, Herfarth et al[9] found oral FMT to be safe and well-tolerated; however, engraftment was largely not achieved, and no clinical benefit was detected.

Consistent with existing studies for UC, single-dose FMT by NGT provided minimal benefit, with 2 of 8 patients treated demonstrating improved PDAI scores but none achieving clinical remission despite improved microbial diversity and an increased shift toward a donor-like microbiota profile.[2] Indeed, in a large randomized trial of FMT for UC, daily enemas for 4 weeks were required for sustained clinical remission beyond 8 weeks.[12] Together, these data corroborate that, compared with the high efficacy of single-dose NGT FMT for rCDI, multiple administrations of FMT may be required to therapeutically manipulate the complex web of genetic, immunologic, and environmental factors underlying UC and pouchitis.

Engraftment

FMT engraftment is generally regarded as the presence of bacteria in donor and post-FMT stool samples that were not present prior to FMT in the recipient. Although it is hypothesized, there is not strong evidence demonstrating that engraftment is required for clinically improved pouchitis, leaving it difficult to predict which subset of patients may benefit from this therapy. Lack of similarity between donor microbiome profiles and recipients post-FMT were noted in both clinically negative and positive studies, suggesting that engraftment may not be associated with clinical benefit, although

Table 10.2.2-1. Fecal Microbiota Transplantation for the Treatment of Pouchitis

Author (Year)	Study Design	No. of Patients	Pouchitis Type	Previous Antibiotic Exposure	Years Since IPAA
Landy et al (2015)[5]	Case series	8	CP	NR	11.3 (4-22)[a]
Stallmach et al (2016)[6]	Case series	5	CARP	Yes, variable	3.8 (1-6)[a]
Fang et al (2016)[7]	Case report	1	CARP	Yes, variable	1
Lan et al (2017)[8]	Case series	13	CP + CDI	Yes, variable	NR
Herfarth et al (2019)[9]	Blinded, placebo-controlled pilot study	6 (4 treatment; 2 placebo)	ADP	Yes, variable	5.7 (1-10)[a]
Selvig et al (2019)[10]	Open-label pilot study	19	CP	42% (8/19) pretreated with rifaximin	6.5 (4-13)[c]
Nishida et al (2019)[11]	Case series	3	CP	NR	7.2[a] (5-9)

Abbreviations: ADP = able to achieve remission with antibiotics, but with flares when weaned; CARP = chronic antibiotic-refractory pouchitis (symptoms persistent despite 3+ trials of ciprofloxacin/flagyl); CP = chronic pouchitis (PDAI > 7 [and 4 weeks of subjective symptoms in Selvig et al[10]]); FCP = fecal calprotectin; FU = follow-up; mPDAI = modified Pouchitis Disease Activity Index, with maximum score of 12 and pouchitis at ≥ 5; NR = not reported; PDAI = Pouchitis Disease Activity Index, with maximum score of 18 and pouchitis at ≥ 7; SAEs = serious adverse events.

Table 10.2.2-1. Fecal Microbiota Transplantation for the Treatment of Pouchitis

FMT	FU	Average PDAI		Average FCP		SAEs
		Before FMT	After FMT	Before FMT	After FMT	
1 FMT via NGT; patient-selected donor	4 weeks	11.5 (10-14)[a]	10.5 (9-14)[a]	NR	NR	None
1-7 FMT via pouchoscopy	12 weeks	10.8 (9-14)[a]	3.8 (2-7)[a]	631	60	None
1 FMT via pouchoscopy	12 weeks	10[b]	0	NR	NR	None
Variable (FMT via pouchoscopy, gastroscopy, enema)	Variable	2.5 (0-6)[a,b]	1.6 (0-4)[a,b]	NR	NR	None
1 FMT via pouchoscopy, then FMT capsules for 14	2 weeks	0.67 (0-1)[a,b]	2.33 (2-3)[a,b]	131	341	None
1 to 2 FMT via pouchoscopy	4 weeks	7 (6-8)[c]	6 (5.5-7.5)[c]	344[c]	240[c]	None
1 FMT via pouchoscopy	8 weeks	12.0 (9-15)[a]	9.3 (7-14)[a]	NR	NR	None

[a]Mean, range.
[b]mPDAI scales used.
[c]Median, interquartile range.

differences in microbiome analysis may confound this statement.[6,10] These discrepant findings beg the question whether the pouch microenvironment has distinct factors precluding engraftment and whether engraftment is necessary for positive clinical outcome.

Summary

Despite uncertainty regarding optimized protocols, optimal donor selection, and potential for inducing remission or maintenance of pouchitis, FMT appears to be safe and well-tolerated. No significant adverse events attributable to FMT in pouchitis have been described, and symptoms like flatulence, mild abdominal pain, and fatigue have been self-limited. Given the small sample size and variable patient populations in current trials, future studies should investigate the ideal dosing regimen and markers predicting FMT response, given the poor associations noted thus far with engraftment. Finally, FMT may have a promising role in clinical symptom management for pouchitis alongside other targeted therapies.

References

1. Shah H, Zezos P. Pouchitis: diagnosis and management. *Curr Opin Gastroenterol.* 2020;36(1):41-47.
2. Ribaldone DG, Resegotti A, Astegiano M. The therapy of chronic pouchitis. *Minerva Gastroenterol Dietol.* 2019;65(4):265-267.
3. Paramsothy S, Paramsothy R, Rubin DT, et al. Faecal microbiota transplantation for inflammatory bowel disease: a systematic review and meta-analysis. *J Crohns Colitis.* 2017;11(10):1180-1199.
4. Zella GC, Hait EJ, Glavan T, et al. Distinct microbiome in pouchitis compared to healthy pouches in ulcerative colitis and familial adenomatous polyposis. *Inflamm Bowel Dis.* 2011;17(5):1092-1100.
5. Landy J, Walker AW, Li JV, et al. Variable alterations of the microbiota, without metabolic or immunological change, following faecal microbiota transplantation in patients with chronic pouchitis. *Sci Rep.* 2015;5:12955.
6. Stallmach A, Lange K, Buening J, et al. Fecal microbiota transfer in patients with chronic antibiotic-refractory pouchitis. *Am J Gastroenterol.* 2016;111(3):441-443.
7. Fang S, Kraft CS, Dhere T, et al. Successful treatment of chronic pouchitis utilizing fecal microbiota transplantation (FMT): a case report. *Int J Color Dis.* 2016;5:1093-1094. doi:10.1007/s00384-015-2428-y
8. Lan N, Ashburn J, Shen B. Fecal microbiota transplantation for *Clostridium difficile* infection in patients with ileal pouches. *Gastroenterol Rep (Oxf).* 2017;5(3):200-207.
9. Herfarth H, Barnes EL, Long MD, et al. Combined endoscopic and oral fecal microbiota transplantation in patients with antibiotic-dependent pouchitis: low clinical efficacy due to low donor microbial engraftment. *Inflamm Intest Dis.* 2019;4(1):1-6.

10. Selvig D, Piceno Y, Terdiman J, et al. Fecal microbiota transplantation in pouchitis: clinical, endoscopic, histologic, and microbiota results from a pilot study. *Dig Dis Sci.* 2020;65(4):1099-1106.
11. Nishida A, Imaeda H, Inatomi O, Bamba S, Sugimoto M, Andoh A. The efficacy of fecal microbiota transplantation for patients with chronic pouchitis: a case series. *Clin Case Rep.* 2019;7(4):782-788.
12. Paramsothy S, Kamm MA, Kaakoush NO, et al. Multidonor intensive faecal microbiota transplantation for active ulcerative colitis: a randomised placebo-controlled trial. *Lancet.* 2017;389(10075):1218-1228.
13. Moayyedi P, Surette MG, Kim PT, et al. Fecal microbiota transplantation induces remission in patients with active ulcerative colitis in a randomized controlled trial. *Gastroenterology.* 2015;149(1):102-109.e6.
14. Steinhart AH, Hiruki T, Brzezinski A, Baker JP. Treatment of left-sided ulcerative colitis with butyrate enemas: a controlled trial. *Aliment Pharmacol Ther.* 1996;10(5):729-736.

10.2

10.2.3 The Role of Fecal Microbiota Transplantation in the Treatment of Irritable Bowel Syndrome

Neena Malik, MD, MSc and
Olga C. Aroniadis, MD, MSc

IBS is a chronic functional bowel disorder characterized by abdominal pain and altered bowel habits. IBS is the most commonly diagnosed GI condition, affecting 10% to 15% of the US population.[1] There are 3 subtypes of IBS, classified by predominant stool form and frequency: diarrhea predominant (IBS-D), constipation predominant (IBS-C), and mixed (IBS-M). The chronicity of IBS and its overlap with a number of other functional disorders result in both impaired quality of life and high health care costs. The pathogenesis of IBS remains unclear, which has created challenges in the development of effective therapeutic strategies. Among other factors, alterations of the intestinal microbiota may play a role in symptom propagation in a subset of IBS patients. This has led to the hypothesis that manipulation of the intestinal microbiota could result in therapeutic benefit for patients with IBS. FMT has emerged as a potential treatment option for IBS due to its ability to alter the intestinal microbiota. However, FMT is not permissible for the treatment of IBS without an approved Investigational New Drug (IND) application through the FDA. Accordingly, FMT has been explored in clinical trials for the treatment of IBS. In this section, we will review the available clinical trial data on the use of FMT in patients with IBS.

Allegretti JR, Kassam Z, eds. *The 6 Ds of Fecal Microbiota Transplantation: A Primer from Decision to Discharge and Beyond* (pp 132-141).
© 2021 SLACK Incorporated.

To date, there have been 6 randomized clinical trials that have investigated the role of FMT for the treatment of IBS (Table 10.2.3-1).[2-7] Broadly, the results have been complex, with 3 randomized clinical trials showing clinical improvement among patients treated with FMT compared with placebo recipients[2,3,7] and the remaining 3 displaying more inconsistent results.[4-6] One study found that a single colonoscopic FMT was associated with improved symptom severity among IBS patients at 3-month follow-up as compared with autologous FMT; however, this improvement was not sustained at 12-month follow-up.[2] A second randomized clinical trial showed symptom improvement in patients with IBS and predominant abdominal bloating receiving nasojejunal FMT as compared with the placebo group at 12 weeks.[3] A third trial reported no difference in symptom severity in patients of varying IBS subtypes receiving colonoscopic FMT with donor stool vs autologous stool.[5] A fourth study showed no significant difference in IBS symptoms between patients receiving FMT capsules for 3 consecutive days vs placebo at 12 weeks.[6] A fifth trial demonstrated that placebo had higher efficacy than FMT capsules in reducing IBS symptoms.[4] Additionally, a meta-analysis of FMT for IBS reported no significant difference in global improvement of IBS symptoms at 12 weeks in FMT vs placebo.[8]

Most recently, El-Salhy et al[7] reported on the largest randomized clinical trial (N = 165) using FMT in the treatment of IBS to help resolve previous contradictory results. Patients with moderate-to-severe IBS (all types) were randomized 1:1:1 to placebo (autologous FMT, own stool), low-dose FMT (30 g), or high-dose FMT (60 g), all by gastroscope. The primary outcome was defined as a clinical response (reduction in IBS symptoms severity score by 50 or more points) at 3 months. Clinical response occurred in 23.6% in the placebo arm, 76.9% in the low-dose FMT arm ($P < .0001$), and 89.1% in the high-dose FMT arm ($P < .0001$) without any related serious adverse events. Despite the strong clinical results from the latest randomized clinical trial, it is difficult to formulate firm conclusions regarding the effectiveness of FMT for IBS due to these heterogeneous results and the paucity of data; however, FMT has promise, and, importantly, there are no concerning safety signals (Figure 10.2.3-1).

Table 10.2.3-1. Randomized Clinical Trials of Fecal Microbiota Transplantation for the Treatment of Irritable Bowel Syndrome

Authors (Year)	Country	Diagnostic Criteria and IBS Subtype	FMT and Control Arms
Johnsen et al (2018)[2]	Norway	Rome III criteria; 53.0% IBS-D, 47.0% IBS-M	• FMT: Donor material (fresh or frozen), 50 to 80 g • Control: Autologous material (participant's own stool)
Holvoet et al (2018)[3]	Belgium	Rome III criteria; predominant IBS with severe abdominal bloating	• FMT: Donor material (fresh), stool grams NR, 2 donors with high microbial richness • Control: Autologous material
Halkjær et al (2018)[4]	Denmark	Rome III criteria; 33.3% IBS-C, 29.4% IBS-D, 37.3% IBS-M	• FMT: Donor material (frozen), 50 g • Control: Placebo

Abbreviations: IBS-SSS = Irritable Bowel Syndrome-Symptom Severity Score; NR = not reported.

Table 10.2.3-1. Randomized Clinical Trials of Fecal Microbiota Transplantation for the Treatment of Irritable Bowel Syndrome

Route of Administration	Sample Size	Follow-Up	Endpoints
Colonoscopy (single administration)	86 (2:1 randomization)	12 weeks	• Clinical outcome: Decrease in IBS-SSS by ≥ 75 points • Microbiome outcome: NR
Nasojejunal tube (single administration)	64 (2:1 randomization)	12 weeks	• Clinical outcome: Self-reported improvement in overall IBS symptoms and abdominal bloating • Microbiome outcome: NR
Capsules (25 capsules daily × 12 days)	52	12 weeks	• Clinical outcome: Decrease in IBS-SSS by ≥ 50 points • Microbiome outcome: Increased diversity in FMT arm vs control

(continued)

Table 10.2.3-1 (continued). Randomized Clinical Trials of Fecal Microbiota Transplantation for the Treatment of Irritable Bowel Syndrome

Authors (Year)	Country	Diagnostic Criteria and IBS Subtype	FMT and Control Arms
Holster et al (2019)[5]	Sweden	Rome III criteria; 25.0% IBS-C, 56.2% IBS-D, 18.8% IBS-M	• FMT: Donor material (frozen), 30 g • Control: Autologous material
Aroniadis et al (2019)[6]	United States	Rome III criteria; 100% IBS-D	• FMT: Donor material (frozen), ~0.38 g/capsule • Control: Placebo (with crossover)

Table 10.2.3-1. Randomized Clinical Trials of Fecal Microbiota Transplantation for the Treatment of Irritable Bowel Syndrome

Route of Administration	Sample Size	Follow-Up	Endpoints
Colonoscopy (single administration)	17	8 weeks	• Clinical outcome: Decrease in Gastrointestinal Symptom Rating Scale–IBS of ≥ 30% • Microbiome outcome: Microbial diversity was not significantly affected by FMT or control
Capsules (25 capsules daily × 3 days)	48	12 weeks	• Clinical outcome: Decrease in IBS-SSS by ≥ 50 points • Microbiome outcomes: FMT responders more likely to exhibit higher ratios of *Bacteroidetes* to Firmicutes at baseline

(continued)

Table 10.2.3-1 (continued). Randomized Clinical Trials of Fecal Microbiota Transplantation for the Treatment of Irritable Bowel Syndrome

Authors (Year)	Country	Diagnostic Criteria and IBS Subtype	FMT and Control Arms
El-Salhy et al (2020)[7]	Norway	Rome IV criteria; 38% IBS-D, 38% IBS-C, 24% IBS-M	• FMT: Donor material (frozen), 30- and 60-g arms, single donor • Control: Autologous material

Inconsistency in results among prior studies is likely due to differences in trial designs. The trials mentioned previously have sample sizes ranging from 16 to 165 study participants, which limits generalizability. In addition, randomized clinical trials have included patients with various IBS subtypes; some trials included patients with any IBS subtype,[4,5] whereas others solely include patients with IBS-D[6] or IBS-D with IBS-M.[2,3] The variability in inclusion criteria between studies with regard to IBS subtype, duration of symptoms, and baseline microbial profiles likely explains some of the differences in study outcomes. The preparation, composition, and amount of donor stool infused and the route of FMT administration (colonoscopy, nasojejunal tube, gastroscope, and capsules) also differ among trials. In reference to composition and storage, the studies that favored FMT used fresh stool[2,3] as opposed to frozen stool, which was used in studies that favored placebo.[4,6] Additionally, the trials that favored FMT used fecal material from a single donor[2,3] as opposed to multiple donors, which was used in a trial that favored placebo.[4] Regarding method of FMT administration, gastroscope, nasojejunal tube,[3] and colonoscopy[2,5] proved more

Table 10.2.3-1. Randomized Clinical Trials of Fecal Microbiota Transplantation for the Treatment of Irritable Bowel Syndrome			
Route of Administration	**Sample Size**	**Follow-Up**	**Endpoints**
Gastroscope (single administration)	165 (1:1:1 randomization: 60 g, 30 g, placebo)	12 weeks	• Clinical outcome: Decrease in IBS-SSS by ≥ 50 points • Microbiome outcomes: FMT responders had higher signals for *Eubacterium biforme*, *Lactobacillus* spp and *Alistipes* spp after FMT and lower signals for *Bacteroides* spp

successful with symptom improvement as compared with capsules.[4,6] FMT dosing is also variable between studies, with some studies giving a single FMT dose[2,3,5] and others giving daily doses for 3 days[6] or 12 days.[4] It has been suggested that maintenance FMT given weekly over the course of 8 weeks, similar to regimens used in prior FMT trials for UC, could prove more efficacious; however, this requires further study. Despite some positive results, there is insufficient evidence to support the use of FMT in clinical practice for patients with IBS.

Summary

Given that currently available treatments for IBS are only modestly effective, there is a strong need for alternate therapeutic options. The intestinal microbiota may be a potential therapeutic target for IBS. Manipulation of the microbiome is possible with FMT, and FMT has been shown to be safe and feasible in patients with IBS.[2-6] However, additional studies investigating patient characteristics and FMT dosing

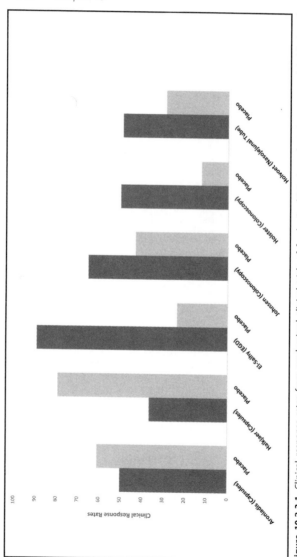

Figure 10.2.3-1. Clinical response rates from randomized clinical trials of fecal microbiota transplantation to treat irritable bowel syndrome. Note: Definitions and eligibility criteria vary by study.[2-7] (EGD = esophagogastroduodenoscopy.)

regimens and delivery methods are needed to better understand the efficacy of FMT for IBS. Much of this work may lie in choosing recipients based on baseline microbial profiles, which may predict response to FMT.[6] Moreover, investigating differences in outcomes among IBS patients who receive single vs maintenance FMT infusions may provide additional insight. Given the uncertainty surrounding the efficacy of FMT for IBS, further studies are needed to develop a more definitive understanding of the role of FMT for IBS, with specific attention to the ideal recipient, FMT dosing regimen, and method of FMT administration.

References

1. Drossman DA, Hasler WL. Rome IV–functional GI disorders: disorders of gut-brain interaction. *Gastroenterology*. 2016;150(6):1257-1261.

2. Johnsen PH, Hilpüsch F, Cavanagh JP, et al. Faecal microbiota transplantation versus placebo for moderate-to-severe irritable bowel syndrome: a double-blind, randomized, placebo-controlled, parallel-group, single-centre trial. *Lancet Gastroenterol Hepatol*. 2018;3(1):17-24.

3. Holvoet T, Joossens M, Jerina B, et al. Fecal microbiota transplantation in irritable bowel syndrome with predominant abdominal bloating: results from a double blind, placebo-controlled clinical trial. *Gastroenterology*. 2018;154(6):S130.

4. Holster S, Brummer RJ, Repsilber D, König J. Fecal microbiota transplantation in irritable bowel syndrome and a randomized placebo-controlled trial. *Gastroenterology*. 2017;152(5):S101-S102.

5. Aroniadis OC, Brandt LJ, Oneto C, et al. Faecal microbiota transplantation for diarrhea-predominant irritable bowel syndrome: a double-blind, randomized, placebo-controlled trial. *Lancet Gastroenterol Hepatol*. 2019;4(9):675-685.

6. Halkjær SI, Christensen AH, Lo BZS, et al. Faecal microbiota transplantation alters gut microbiota in patients with irritable bowel syndrome: results from a randomized, double-blind placebo-controlled study. *Gut*. 2018;67(12):2107-2115.

7. El-Salhy M, Hatlebakk JG, Gilja OH, Kristoffersen AB, Hausken T. Efficacy of faecal microbiota transplantation for patients with irritable bowel syndrome in a randomised, double-blind, placebo-controlled study. *Gut*. 2020;69(5):859-867.

8. Xu D, Chen VL, Steiner CA, et al. Efficacy of fecal microbiota transplantation in irritable bowel syndrome: a systematic review and meta-analysis. *Am J Gastroenterol*. 2019;114(7):1043-1050.

10.3

The Role of Fecal Microbiota Transplantation in the Treatment of Liver Diseases

*Chathur Acharya, MD and
Jasmohan S. Bajaj, MD, MS*

With the emerging role of the gut microbiome in gastroenterology and liver disease, there has been a substantial interest in using FMT in hepatology as a potential therapeutic intervention. Over the past 5 years there have been promising data generated to support this avenue, and there are many more studies underway. The FDA has not approved FMT as a therapeutic option for chronic liver disease. This section will examine current and emerging data for FMT in different liver conditions.

Preclinical Evidence for Fecal Microbiota Transplantation in Liver Disease

There have been investigations into the use of FMT to treat liver disease in rodent models. Zhou et al[1] reported a study of autologous FMT daily for 8 weeks in mice with high-fat diet–induced nonalcoholic fatty

Allegretti JR, Kassam Z, eds. *The 6 Ds of Fecal
Microbiota Transplantation: A Primer From
Decision to Discharge and Beyond* (pp 142-148).
© 2021 SLACK Incorporated.

liver disease (NAFLD)/nonalcoholic steatohepatitis (NASH) and demonstrated that FMT improved steatohepatitis and systemic inflammation. Another study in acute liver failure–related hepatic encephalopathy demonstrated that duodenally infused FMT daily for 3 weeks resulted in improved behavior, memory, and learning and reduced systemic inflammation.[2] This study was limited by the lack of microbiome assessments pre- and post-FMT.[2] In alcoholic liver disease models, when FMT was performed with FMT material from alcohol-resistant donor mice, FMT restored the intestinal microbiota composition to that of the donor mice. Additionally, the treatment prevented alcohol-induced gut barrier changes and also prevented the development of liver disease related to alcohol.[3] Overall, preclinical work suggests that FMT is a promising intervention for various microbiome-mediated liver diseases.

Fecal Microbiota Transplantation Clinical Trials in Humans

Given the promising preclinical work, a number of investigators have begun to examine to role of FMT in humans with various liver diseases.

Primary Sclerosing Cholangitis

Primary sclerosing cholangitis (PSC) is a rare, progressive cholestatic liver disease, notable for leading to bile duct strictures, and often linked with IBD. Currently, no FDA- or European Medicines Agency (EMA)–approved therapies exist for this indication, and patients may ultimately require liver transplantation. Allegretti et al[4] conducted a Phase 1b pilot open-label study of 10 patients with early-stage PSC with concomitant IBD. Patients underwent a single FMT by colonoscopy (90 mL) from a single healthy donor. The primary objective was safety and feasibility. The treatment was well-tolerated, and no patients experienced a treatment-related serious adverse event. Overall, 30% (3/10) of patients had improvement of 50% or greater alkaline phosphatase levels, a key biliary biomarker in PSC. Microbial diversity of the patients resembled the donor within 1 week and was sustained through the end of the study (6 months).[4] Given the unmet medical need for this disease, FMT remains a promising therapy and requires further study (Figure 10.3-1).

Alcoholic Hepatitis

Alcoholic hepatitis is characterized by inflammation in the liver post-excessive alcohol consumption. It has been suggested that alcohol consumption can lead to dysbiosis, and this alteration of the gut microbiome may propagate the disease.

In a study of patients with severe alcoholic hepatitis, FMT was compared with other standard-of-care (SOC) interventions. Among 51 patients enrolled, 16 were treated with FMT. Overall, patients who received FMT had the highest survival rates at 1 and 3 months. Specifically, the proportions of patients surviving at the end of 1 and 3 months in the steroids, nutrition, pentoxifylline, and FMT arms were 63%, 47%, 40%, and 75% ($P=.179$) and 38%, 29%, 30%, and 75% ($P=.036$), respectively. Following FMT, significant beneficial changes in the microbiome were noted.

A number of studies, including randomized clinical trials, are actively recruiting at the time of writing (NCT03091010 [open label, nasojejunal], NCT03827772 [open label, nasojejunal], and NCT03416751 [randomized clinical trial, enema]). These studies highlight the interest in and promise of FMT in alcoholic hepatitis.

Nonalcoholic Fatty Liver Disease and Nonalcoholic Steatohepatitis

NAFLD is characterized by fat deposition or hepatic steatosis (> 5%) without secondary causes. It is often associated with other metabolic conditions, such as diabetes mellitus, obesity, and metabolic syndrome. NASH is separately defined as the presence of at least 5% hepatic steatosis with inflammation and the addition of hepatocyte injury with or without fibrosis.[5] This can progress to cirrhosis and has become the leading cause of liver transplantation in the United States. There are no FDA- or EMA-approved therapies currently. Given the promising preclinical data previously described, there is interest in the use of FMT to restore the microbiome in patients with NAFLD/NASH.

Xue et al[6] reported a pilot placebo-controlled trial (N = 47) of FMT in NAFLD. The primary outcome assessed was change in fat attenuation parameter assessed by FibroTouch. They demonstrated that patients in the FMT arm had significant reduction in fat attenuation parameter compared with the control group. Specifically, the FMT arm had a mean decrease of 9.26 ± 29.31 compared with an increase of 12.21 ± 24.48 in the control arm ($P=.038$).[6]

Parvathy et al[7] performed a pilot randomized clinical trial using FMT via upper endoscopy compared with autologous FMT in patients

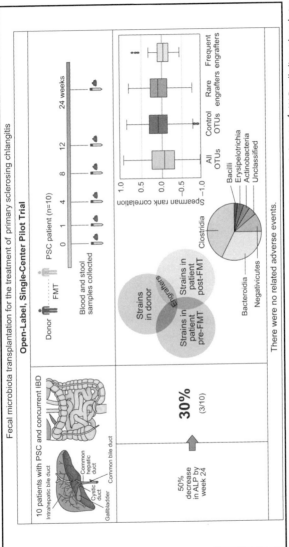

Figure 10.3-1. Fecal microbiota transplantation for the treatment of primary sclerosing cholangitis.[4] (ALP = alkaline phosphate; OTU = operational taxonomical unit.)

with NAFLD. Overall, they did not report any related serious adverse events and demonstrated improvement in small intestinal permeability biomarkers.[7]

At the time of writing, there are several other studies underway (NCT02469272, NCT02721264, and NCT03803540). The use of FMT for NASH/NAFLD appears to be a promising intervention given the lack of viable medically options for this large patient population. Further discussion of NAFLD can be found in Chapter 10.6: "The Role of Fecal Microbiota Transplantation in the Treatment of Obesity, Metabolic Syndrome, and Nonalcoholic Fatty Liver Disease."

Recurrent Overt Hepatic Encephalopathy

Overt hepatic encephalopathy (OHE) is a clinical sequela of decompensated liver cirrhosis. This clinical symptom is often treated and prevented with antibiotics and/or lactulose, giving rise to the interest in microbial manipulations for this clinical condition.

Two randomized clinical trials assessing the use of FMT for the prevention of recurrent OHE have been completed.[8,9] The first trial treated 20 patients with recurrent OHE on maximum medical therapy (rifaximin and lactulose) and included treatment with preprocedure antibiotics followed by enema FMT compared with SOC (Figure 10.3-2).[8] The second trial assessed the same patient population but treated with FMT capsules alone vs placebo without pretreatment antibiotics.[9] Both studies were Phase 1b conducted under an FDA IND application. One donor with high relative abundance of *Lachnospiraceae* and *Ruminococcaceae* was used in each study. Overall, both studies showed safety, engraftment of the FMT material, improvement in cognitive function, and improvement in clinical outcomes. Patients in the first trial who received FMT via enema had sustained improvement in their outcomes for more than 1 year post-therapy.[8]

Moreover, when stool from OHE patients were introduced in germ-free mice, it induced neuroinflammation and microglial activation, which resolved after stools post-FMT were used for colonization of germ-free mice.[10]

There are a number of studies underway for FMT in OHE (NCT03420482 [capsules], NCT03439982 [colonoscopy]), as well as a Phase 2 randomized clinical trials using both oral and rectal enema route of FMT (NCT03796598).

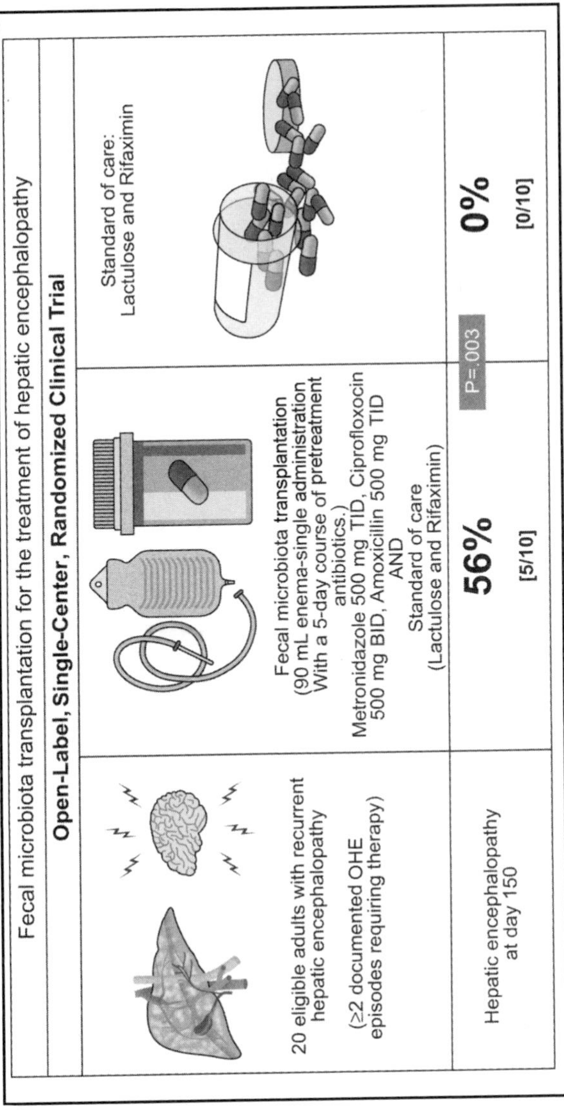

Figure 10.3-2. Fecal microbiota transplantation for the treatment of overt hepatic encephalopathy.[8] (BID = 2 times/day; TID = 3 times/day.)

Summary

The gut-liver axis has emerged as a promising area of research. Pilot data suggests there may be a role for FMT in PSC, which does not have any approved therapies. Preliminary studies also suggest the role of FMT in alcoholic hepatitis and NAFLD/NASH with a number of ongoing studies in both diseases. Lastly, there are 2 randomized clinical trials that show compelling data for the role of FMT in recurrent OHE with sustained improvement in clinical outcomes more than 1 year following therapy. Overall, there is potential for microbiome therapeutics to unlock new medicine for patients suffering from a range of liver diseases.

References

1. Zhou D, Pan Q, Shen F, et al. Total fecal microbiota transplantation alleviates high-fat diet-induced steatohepatitis in mice via beneficial regulation of gut microbiota. *Sci Rep.* 2017;7(1):1529.
2. Wang WW, Zhang Y, Huang XB, You N, Zheng L, Li J. Fecal microbiota transplantation prevents hepatic encephalopathy in rats with carbon tetrachloride-induced acute hepatic dysfunction. *World J Gastroenterol.* 2017;23(38):6983-6994.
3. Ferrere G, Wrzosek L, Cailleux F, et al. Fecal microbiota manipulation prevents dysbiosis and alcohol-induced liver injury in mice. *J Hepatol.* 2017;66(4):806-815.
4. Allegretti JR, Kassam Z, Carrellas M, et al. Fecal microbiota transplantation in patients with primary sclerosing cholangitis: a pilot clinical trial. *Am J Gastroenterol.* 2019;114(7):1071-1079.
5. Vilstrup H, Amodio P, Bajaj J, et al. Hepatic encephalopathy in chronic liver disease: 2014 Practice Guideline by the American Association for the Study of Liver Diseases and the European Association for the Study of the Liver. *Hepatology.* 2014;60(2):715-735.
6. Xue LF, Luo WH, Wu LH, He XX, Xia HHX, Chen Y. Fecal microbiota transplantation for the treatment of nonalcoholic fatty liver disease. *Explor Res Hypothesis Med.* 2019;4(1):12-18.
7. Parvathy SN, Beaton MD, Medding J, et al. Su1553–Impact of fecal microbial transplantation on intestinal permeability in non alcoholic fatty liver disease. *Gastroenterology.* 2018;154(6 suppl 1):S1176-S1177.
8. Bajaj JS, Kassam Z, Fagan A, et al. Fecal microbiota transplant from a rational stool donor improves hepatic encephalopathy: a randomized clinical trial. *Hepatology.* 2017;66(6):1727-1738.
9. Bajaj JS, Salzman NH, Acharya C, et al. Fecal microbial transplant capsules are safe in hepatic encephalopathy: a Phase 1, randomized, placebo-controlled trial. *Hepatology.* 2019;70(5):1690-1703.
10. Liu R, Kang JD, Sartor RB, et al. Neuroinflammation in murine cirrhosis is dependent on the gut microbiome and is attenuated by fecal transplant. *Hepatology.* 2020;71(2):611-626.

10.4

The Role of Fecal Microbiota Transplantation in the Treatment of Autism Spectrum Disorder

*Thomas J. Borody, MD, PhD, DSc and
Anoja W. Gunaratne, BAMS (Hon), MSc, PhD*

Autism spectrum disorder (ASD) encompasses a heterogeneous group of child neurodevelopment conditions characterized by disorders in social interaction, verbal and nonverbal communication, sensory processing, and repetitive behaviors.[1] In a 2014 report by the Centers for Disease Control and Prevention (CDC), the prevalence of ASD among 8-year-old children was found to have increased by 15% over the prior 2 years, resulting in 1 in 59 children having ASD.[2] In up to 50% of children with ASD, development occurs typically until approximately 2 years of age, at which time regression and loss of previously acquired communication and social skills occurs.[3,4] Treatment options are limited and include behavioral therapy, speech-language and/or social therapy, psychiatric medications for a specific cohort, and dietary and nutritional approaches.[5] However, no treatments currently exist that target the underlying etiology or core symptoms of ASD.

Allegretti JR, Kassam Z, eds. *The 6 Ds of Fecal Microbiota Transplantation: A Primer From Decision to Discharge and Beyond* (pp 149-157).
© 2021 SLACK Incorporated.

Link Between the Gut Microbiome and Autism Spectrum Disorder

Although the etiopathogenesis of ASD remains unknown, increasing evidence suggests that the gut microbiome plays a pivotal role in the development and perpetuation of ASD symptoms. Prenatal and early-life antibiotic exposure are associated with an increased risk of ASD development.[6,7] Recent evidence suggests that children with ASD have abnormal gut microbiome composition (dysbiosis), including increased levels of *Clostridia, Lactobacillus, Collinsella, Corynebacterium,* and *Dorea* and decreased *Bacteroidetes, Alistipes, Bilophila, Dialister, Parabacteroides,* and *Veillonella* species.[8] Finegold et al[9,10] demonstrated the presence of abnormal *Clostridia* and *Desulfovibrio* bacteria in the stool of children with ASD compared with controls. They postulated that neurotoxins manufactured by these pathogens are capable, either via circulation or by neuronal streaming, of crossing the blood-brain barrier to cause ASD-like symptoms. It has been demonstrated that children with ASD experience significantly higher rates of GI symptoms compared with healthy controls, including higher rates of diarrhea, constipation, and abdominal pain.[11] Further, the severity of GI symptoms has been shown to positively correlate with disease severity, strengthening the link between a gut-brain connection in ASD.[11] This section will review the current literature assessing the use of microbiome interventions, including FMT, in patients with ASD.

Manipulation of the Gut Microbiome in Autism Spectrum Disorder

Early studies using antibiotics have resulted in significant, albeit temporary, improvements in ASD symptoms. Vancomycin, one of the first studied antibiotics, is a nonabsorbable agent with broad activity against the dominant phyla of obligate anaerobes (*Bacteroidetes* and *Firmicutes*) in the intestine.[12] In a pilot clinical trial that assessed the use of oral vancomycin for 8 weeks in children with ASD, dramatic reversal of ASD symptoms and improvement in gut symptoms were observed in 8 of 10 patients.[13] However, the benefits were lost a few weeks after stopping treatment, pointing to the need for continuing intervention.[12] In another study, 6 months of antibiotics (amoxicillin and/or azithromycin) helped to reduce ASD symptoms and improve behavior.[14]

Clinical studies examining the use of prebiotics and probiotics in ASD treatment have shown mixed effects on ASD symptoms.[15-21] Multiple studies have shown improvements in GI symptoms, irritability scores, concentration, carrying out orders, and behavior after either prebiotics or probiotic supplementation in children with ASD.[15-20] One placebo-controlled study (N = 39) showed lower levels of *Clostridioides* in stools after probiotics (*Lactobacillus plantarum*) supplementation; however, no major differences in behavior or GI symptoms were observed.[22]

More recently, FMT has been used as a treatment for ASD, with promising results (Table 10.4-1).[23-26] A number of methods have been used to administer FMT to adults and children, including raw, homogenized, and filtered fresh FMT material and lyophilized FMT material (encapsulated or as powder) to facilitate delivery to the entire GI tract.[27,28] In an open-label study conducted in 18 children with ASD, FMT for up to 8 weeks led to a 82% reduction in GI symptoms and significant improvements in core ASD symptoms by 22% (language, social interaction, and behavior measured by the validated Childhood Autism Rating Scale) compared with baseline, which corresponded with increased microbial diversity.[24] At 2-year follow-up of these children, most GI symptom improvements were maintained, and ASD-related symptoms further improved at the 2-year review, with 44% of participants below the ASD diagnostic cut-off scores (Figure 10.4-1).[25] After FMT, *Bacteroidetes* and *Firmicutes* increased and *Clostridioides* was inhibited in the GI tract.[24,25] No significant safety concerns were observed, and the treatment was well-tolerated. A limitation of this promising study is that it was uncontrolled with a patient-reported outcome and there was an absence of dose-finding preliminary work to identify the starting dose regimen. Additionally, it is unclear whether pretreatment antibiotics and bowel lavage are required for clinical efficacy. Notably, it took 5 to 6 weeks of daily FMT for GI symptoms to appropriately respond, supporting the role of maintenance therapy. Following this proof-of-principle study, dose and dose-regimen studies are needed, and once the ideal dose regimen is identified, placebo-controlled trials are warranted.

Table 10.4-1. Fecal Microbiota Transplantation for the Treatment of Autism Spectrum Disorder

Authors (Year)	Country	Design	Population	Pretreatment Antibiotics	Bowel Lavage
Ward et al (2016)[23]	Canada	Case series	8 children and 1 adult with ASD	Oral vancomycin (40 mg/kg/day divided BID for 7 days) with or without nitazoxanide (300 mg BID), colistin (37 mg BID), nystatin (500,000 units TID) each for 7 days	Yes
Kang et al (2017)[24] and Kang et al (2019)[25]	United States	Open-label pilot study	18 children with ASD and GI problems	Oral vancomycin (40 mg/kg/day divided TID for 14 days)	Yes

In Practice: The Australian Experience

Currently, at the Centre for a Digestive Disease in New South Wales, Australia, children with ASD are treated with a minimum 12 weeks of combination antibiotics to reduce the microbiota in the gut and systemic toxin exposure. This is followed by treatment with encapsulated FMT to restore the microbiome in the GI tract. Approximately 60 children have been treated with this protocol, with promising results and no safety concerns (unpublished data).

Table 10.4-1. Fecal Microbiota Transplantation for the Treatment of Autism Spectrum Disorder

PPI	FMT Induction	FMT Maintenance	Outcome	Follow-Up	Comments
NR	FMT capsules (n = 12 to 24) on Day 0	FMT enema (300 to 400 mL, 50 to 100 g) on Days 0 and 1	Safety, clinical symptoms, and microbiome profile	Variable	Well-tolerated and no SAEs; marked clinical improvement in pediatric patients; microbiome analysis suggested *Bacteroides*, *Barnesiella*, *Parabacteroides*, *Sutterella*, *Parasutterella*, *Clostridiales*, and *Erysipetotrichales* were most altered
Yes	FMT oral (2.5 × 10^{12} cells/day for 2 days divided into 3 daily doses) orFMT enema (2.5 × 10^{12} cells/day—single	FMT oral (2.5 × 10^9 cells/daily for 7 to 8 weeks)	Safety, GI symptoms (GSRS, DSR), ASD symptoms (CARS, PGI-III, ABC, SRS, VABS-II) microbiome profile	8 weeks[24] and 2 years[25]	See Figure 10.4-1 for details *(continued)*

Summary

Studies increasingly implicate the microbiome in the pathophysiology of ASD. These findings are further strengthened by the resolution of GI and behavioral symptoms post-modulation of the gut microbiome with antibiotics, probiotics, and FMT, which have been demonstrated in a proof-of-principle human study. It has been proposed that enteric-derived *Clostridioides* toxin-releasing bacteria capable of producing systemic effects may explain the pathophysiology of ASD, which has some

Table 10.4-1 (continued). Fecal Microbiota Transplantation for the Treatment of Autism Spectrum Disorder

Authors (Year)	Country	Design	Population	Pretreatment Antibiotics	Bowel Lavage
Zhao et al (2019)[26]	China	Open-label randomized wait-list–controlled clinical trial	48 children with ASD	NR	Yes

Abbreviations: ABC = Autism Behavior Checklist; BID = 2 times/day; DSR = daily stool record; GSI = Gastrointestinal Severity Index; GSRS = Gastrointestinal Symptom Rating Scale; NR = not reported; PGI-III = Parent Global Impressions-III; PPI = proton-pump inhibitor; SAE = serious adverse event; SRS = Social Responsiveness Scale; TID = 3 times daily; VABS-II = Vineland Adaptive Behavior Scales, 2nd edition.

clinical support. Given that manipulation of the colonic microbiota can markedly improve ASD symptoms as well as concurrent GI symptoms, FMT for ASD warrants further investigation into its efficacy and safety.

Acknowledgment

The authors acknowledge Dr. Annabel Clancy, Research Manager at the Centre for Digestive Diseases.

References

1. Masi A, DeMayo MM, Glozier N, Guastella AJ. An overview of spectrum disorder, heterogeneity and treatment options. *Neurosci Bull.* 2017;33(2):183-193.
2. Baio J, Wiggins L, Christiansen DL, et al. Prevalence of autism spectrum disorder among children aged 8 years—Autism and Developmental Disabilities Monitoring Network, 11 sites, United States, 2014. *MMWR Surveill Summ.* 2018;67(No. SS-6):1-23.

Table 10.4-1. Fecal Microbiota Transplantation for the Treatment of Autism Spectrum Disorder

PPI	FMT Induction	FMT Maintenance	Outcome	Follow-Up	Comments
NR	FMT by colonoscopy and gastroscopy on Day 0	FMT by colonoscopy and gastroscopy at Weeks 8 and 16	Safety, GI symptoms (GSI), ASD symptoms (CARS), microbiome profile	8 weeks and 16 weeks	Well-tolerated with no reported SAEs; GSI improvement in FMT arm vs control ($P < .05$); CARS decrease by 10.8% in FMT arm vs 0.8% in control ($P < .001$); FMT shifted microbiome profile to a healthy state and decreased *Bacteroides fragilis*

3.   Baird G, Charman T, Pickles A, et al. Regression, developmental trajectory and associated problems in disorders in the spectrum: the SNAP study. *J Autism Dev Disord*. 2008;38(10):1827-1836.

4.   Ozonoff S, Heung K, Byrd R, Hansen R, Hertz-Picciotto I. The onset of autism: patterns of symptom emergence in the first years of life. *Autism Res*. 2008;1(6):320-328.

5.   Francis K. Autism interventions: a critical update. *Dev Med Child Neurol*. 2005;47(7):493-499.

6.   Niehus R, Lord C. Early medical history of children with autism spectrum disorders. *J Dev Behav Pediatr*. 2006;27(2 Suppl):S120-S127.

7.   Yassour M, Vatanen T, Siljander H, et al. Natural history of the infant gut microbiome and impact of antibiotic treatment on bacterial strain diversity and stability. *Sci Transl Med*. 2016;8(343):343ra81.

8.   Strati F, Cavalieri D, Albanese D, et al. New evidences on the altered gut microbiota in autism spectrum disorders. *Microbiome*. 2017;5(1):24.

9.   Finegold SM, Dowd SE, Gontcharova V, et al. Pyrosequencing study of fecal microflora of autistic and control children. *Anaerobe*. 2010;16(4):444-53.

10. Finegold SM, Molitoris D, Song Y, et al. Gastrointestinal microflora studies in late-onset autism. *Clin Infect Dis*. 2002;35(Suppl 1):S6-16.

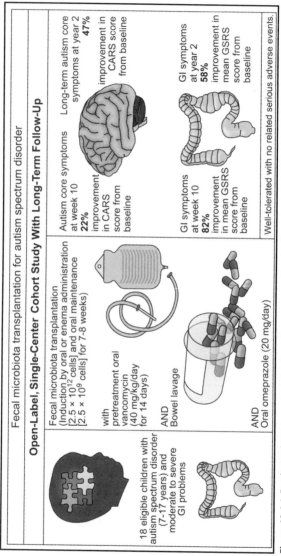

Figure 10.4-1. Fecal microbiota transplantation for autism spectrum disorder.[24]

11. Adams JB, Johansen LJ, Powell LD, Quig D, Rubin RA. Gastrointestinal flora and gastrointestinal status in children with autism—comparisons to typical children and correlation with autism severity. *BMC Gastroenterol.* 2011;11:22.

12. Isaac S, Scher JU, Djukovic A, et al. Short- and long-term effects of oral vancomycin on the human intestinal microbiota. *J Antimicrob Chemother.* 2017;72(1):128-136.

13. Sandler RH, Finegold SM, Bolte ER, et al. Short-term benefit from oral vancomycin treatment of regressive-onset autism. *J Child Neurol.* 2000;15(7):429-435.

14. Kuhn M, Grave S, Bransfield R, Harris S. Long term antibiotic therapy may be an effective treatment for children co-morbid with Lyme disease and autism spectrum disorder. *Med Hypotheses.* 2012;78(5):606-615.

15. Grimaldi R, Gibson GR, Vulevic J, et al. A prebiotic intervention study in children with autism spectrum disorders (ASDs). *Microbiome.* 2018;6(1):133.

16. Sanctuary MR, Kain JN, Chen SY, et al. Pilot study of probiotic/colostrum supplementation on gut function in children with autism and gastrointestinal symptoms. *PLoS One.* 2019;14(1):e0210064.

17. Kałużna-Czaplińska J, Błaszczyk S. The level of arabinitol in autistic children after probiotic therapy. *Nutrition.* 2012;28(2):124-126.

18. Shaaban SY, El Gendy YG, Mehanna NS, et al. The role of probiotics in children with autism spectrum disorder: a prospective, open-label study. *Nutr Neurosci.* 2018;21(9):676-681.

19. Grossi E, Melli S, Dunca D, Terruzzi V. Unexpected improvement in core autism spectrum disorder symptoms after long-term treatment with probiotics. *SAGE Open Med Case Rep.* 2016;4:2050313X16666231.

20. West R, Roberts E, Sichel LS, Sichel J. Improvements in gastrointestinal symptoms among children with autism spectrum disorder receiving the Delpro® probiotic and immunomodulatory formulation. *J Probiotics Health.* 2013;1(1).

21. Tomova A, Husarova V, Lakatosova S, et al. Gastrointestinal microbiota in children with autism in Slovakia. *Physiol Behav.* 2015;138:179-187.

22. Parracho HMRT, Gibson GR, Knott FJ, Bosscher D, Kleerebezem M, Mccartney A. A double-blind, placebo-controlled, crossover-designed probiotic feeding study in children diagnosed with autistic spectrum disorders. *Int J Probiotics Prebiotics.* 2010;5(2):69-74.

23. Ward L, O'Grady H, Wu K, et al. Combined oral fecal capsules plus fecal enema as treatment of late onset autism spectrum disorder in children: report of a small case series, in IDweek (New Orleans, LA:). 2016. Accessed October 22, 2020. https://idsa.confex.com/idsa/2016/webprogram/Paper60261.html

24. Kang DW, Adams JB, Gregory AC, et al. Microbiota transfer therapy alters gut ecosystem and improves gastrointestinal and autism symptoms: an open-label study. *Microbiome.* 2017;5(1):10.

25. Kang DW, Adams JB, Coleman DM, et al. Long-term benefit of microbiota transfer therapy on autism symptoms and gut microbiota. *Sci Rep.* 2019;9(1):5821.

26. Zhao H, Gao X, Xi L, et al. Fecal microbiota transplantation for children with autism spectrum disorder. *Gastrointest Endosc.* 2019;89(6):AB512-AB513.

27. Borody, T.J., Paramsothy, S. & Agrawal, G. Fecal microbiota transplantation: indications, methods, evidence, and future directions. *Curr Gastroenterol Rep.* 2013;15(8):337.

28. Gurram B, Sue PK. Fecal microbiota transplantation in children: current concepts. *Curr Opin Pediatr.* 2019;31(5):623-629.

10.5

The Role of Fecal Microbiota Transplantation in the Decolonization of Antibiotic-Resistant Bacteria

Christopher Saddler, MD and Nasia Safdar, MD, PhD

Antibiotic resistance is a serious worldwide threat, causing more than 2 million infections annually and 23,000 deaths in the United States alone.[1] Furthermore, these infections lead to a significant economic impact, with a median increase in total hospital costs of $38,121 compared with those with antibiotic-susceptible infection.[2] To date, several strategies have been employed to combat antibiotic resistance, primarily based in infection control and antimicrobial stewardship. For those already colonized, the risk of infection and associated morbidity and mortality is increased,[3] yet no optimal strategy exists to address this clinical challenge. Decolonization protocols using antibiotics have had inconsistent outcomes and raise the risk of developing further resistance. Accordingly, this practice cannot be recommended for routine use.[4-9] Given that several studies have demonstrated the efficacy of FMT for preventing recurrence of *Clostridium difficile* infection (CDI; previously *Clostridium difficile* infection) via restoration of the gut microbiome, it has been postulated that FMT may have a role in antibiotic-resistant bacteria (ARB) decolonization. This section highlights the data on decolonization of ARB by FMT.

Allegretti JR, Kassam Z, eds. *The 6 Ds of Fecal Microbiota Transplantation: A Primer From Decision to Discharge and Beyond* (pp 158-168).

The widespread early adoption of FMT for rCDI and the overall increased understanding of the microbiome has sparked significant interest in FMT for ARB decolonization. Initially, as FMT for rCDI became more widely used, case reports and case series began to emerge reporting on concomitant non–*C. difficile* ARB decolonization. Notably, in 2016 Millan et al[10] reported a sustained reduction in antibiotic resistance genes following FMT for rCDI in those with symptom resolution, adding to the proof-of-concept data. Overall, these preliminary results were favorable; however, these studies were limited due to small sample size, study design limitations, and reporting bias. These results are summarized in Table 10.5-1.[11-22]

Patients with rCDI are frequently colonized with vancomycin-resistant *Enterococcus* (VRE), with prevalence nearing 20%.[23] Accordingly, several studies were conducted examining the role of FMT of decolonizing VRE. Dubberke et al[15] reported a 72.7% VRE decolonization rate in a subanalysis of 11 patients from a randomized clinical trial evaluating a microbiome-based therapy for rCDI. Additionally, Santiago et al[22] reported a statistically significant difference between decolonization of VRE comparing allogeneic FMT (FMT from a healthy donor) with autologous FMT (FMT from one's own stool; used as a placebo). After 6 weeks, 92% (11/12) of those initially colonized were decolonized in the group receiving allogenic FMT, whereas only 43% (3/7) of those initially colonized in the group receiving autologous FMT were decolonized.

Other clinical applications regarding ARB have been explored. Tariq et al[19] reported decreased rates of recurrent urinary tract infections (UTIs) and improved antibiotic susceptibility profiles among those who underwent FMT for rCDI and had a history of recurrent UTIs. These data opens the door for other potential studies investigating the role FMT in reestablishing antibiotic susceptibility in locations outside the gut.

With these promising results in the co-colonized CDI population, FMT with the primary purpose of ARB decolonization has been increasingly pursued. Case reports and small case series among patients without concurrent CDI began to emerge, reporting 100% efficacy for decolonization of extended-spectrum beta-lactamase (ESBL)–producing organisms and carbapenem-resistant *Enterobacteriaceae* (CRE).[24-29] Subsequently, larger case series and pilot prospective, uncontrolled studies followed with mixed, but generally promising, results suggesting 37.5% to 87.5% efficacy for ARB decolonization without any safety concerns.[30-36] However, only 1 randomized clinical trial (N=39) by Huttner et al[37] has been reported to date, which showed more modest potential benefit (41% vs 29% decolonization rate of extended-spectrum beta-lactamase *Enterobacteriaceae* and CRE) not

Table 10.5-1. Fecal Microbiota Transplantation for Recurrent *Clostridioides difficile* Infection With Concomitant Antibiotic-Resistant Bacteria

Author (Year)	N	Study Design	Target Organisms	Antibiotic as Prep	Multiple FMT	Decolonization %
Crum-Cianflone et al (2015)[11]	1	CR	MRSA, CRE, VRE, PA	No	No	100
Stripling et al (2015)[12]	1	CR	VRE	No	No	100[a]
Jang et al (2015)[13]	1	CR	VRE	No	Yes	0
García-Fernández et al (2016)[14]	1	CR	CRE	No	No	100
Dubberke et al (2016)[15]	11	Prospective open-label MCT	VRE	No	Yes	72.7
Santiago et al (2019)[16]	9	Prospective open-label MCT	VRE	No	NR	100
Sohn (2016)[17]	3	CS	VRE	No	Yes	0

(continued)

Table 10.5-1 (continued). Fecal Microbiota Transplantation for Recurrent Clostridioides difficile Infection With Concomitant Antibiotic-Resistant Bacteria

Author (Year)	N	Study Design	Target Organisms	Antibiotic as Prep	Multiple FMT	Decolonization %
Innes et al (2017)[18]	1	CR	CRE, ESBL	5 days oral vancomycin and neomycin	No	100
Tariq et al (2017)[19]	8	Retrospective CS	Recurrent UTI	No	No	Reduction in UTI frequency and resistance profiles
Ponte et al (2017)[20]	1	CR	CRE	No	No	100
Wang et al (2018)[21]	1	CR	ESBL, MDR GNR	No	No	100[b]
Santiago et al (2019)[22]	12	Placebo-controlled randomized clinical trial	VRE	No	No	91.7

Abbreviations: CR = case report; CRE = carbapenem-resistant *Enterobacteriaceae*; CS = case series; GNR = gram-negative rod; MCT = multicenter trial; MDR = multidrug-resistant; MRSA = methicillin-resistant *Staphylococcus aureus*; NR = not reported; PA = *Pseudomonas aeruginosa*.

[a]decline in enterococcal relative fecal abundance from 24% to 0.2%; no recurrence of infection.
[b]Clinical resolution; no recurrent UTI after 25-year history with negative urine cultures in 25 months intervening.

meeting statistical significance. This study was unfortunately hampered by not meeting goal sample size and thus lacked statistical power. It also used 5 days of oral antibiotics for intestinal decolonization. Table 10.5-2 summarizes the current data of non-CDI trials.[24-38] Fortunately, numerous studies as reported on clinicaltrials.gov are in progress, which may add to our knowledge base.

The Huttner et al[37] study perfectly demonstrates some of the greater issues in the study of FMT for ARB decolonization. First, the definition of colonization has been widely variable and requires uniformity. Second, the methodology of assessing decolonization must also be determined, with clarification regarding whether use of rectal swabs or stool in selective culture, polymerase chain reaction arrays for antibiotic resistance mechanisms, or more elaborate testing such as stool for metagenomics evaluation of antibiotic resistance genes is most appropriate. Third, the methodology of studies should be standardized, including whether antibiotics are given for intestinal decolonization; whether bowel lavage is performed; and what dose, what frequency, and via what route FMT should be delivered. These require more systematic study moving forward. Further study is also needed to establish factors that predict success or failure of ARB decolonization. Importantly, future studies must be placebo controlled to assess efficacy given that spontaneous decolonization of ARBs does occur, at highly variable rates. In addition, studies must focus on individual organisms as opposed to an aggregation of multiple ARBs, given that there may be variability in effect size. Finally, although FMT appears safe, the long-term safety and efficacy will require comprehensive continued monitoring.

Summary

Overall, FMT for ARB decolonization is an intervention that is in its infancy and requires significant further study to identify the optimal target population. FMT should remain an investigational agent at this point for ARB decolonization until established interventional strategies and randomized controlled trials have determined the benefit.

Table 10.5-2. Fecal Microbiota Transplantation for Antibiotic-Resistant Bacteria Decolonization Without Concomitant *Clostridioides difficile* Infection

Author (Year)	N	Study Design	Target Organisms	Antibiotic as Prep	Multiple FMT	Decolonization %
Freedman & Eppes (2014)[25]	1	CR	CRE	No	No	100
Singh et al (2014)[28]	1	CR	ESBL	No	No	100
Lagier et al (2015)[27]	1	CR	CRE	Oral colomycin 2.5 MIU and gentamicin 100 mg × 4 doses over 24 hours	No	100
Wei (2015)[38]	5	CR	MRSA	Vancomycin 2 g/day for 3 days	Yes	100
Biliński et al (2016)[24]	1	CR	CRE, ESBL	No	No	100
Lahtinen et al (2017)[26]	1	CS	ESBL	No	No	100
Stalenhoef et al (2017)[29]	1	CR	ESBL, CRPA	No	No	ESBL persisted, PA cleared

(continued)

Table 10.5-2 (continued). Fecal Microbiota Transplantation for Antibiotic-Resistant Bacteria Decolonization Without Concomitant *Clostridioides difficile* Infection

Author (Year)	N	Study Design	Target Organisms	Antibiotic as Prep	Multiple FMT	Decolonization %
Biliński et al (2017)[31]	20	Prospective, open-label, unblinded, uncontrolled, single-center	CRE, ESBL, CRPA, VRE, ACTB, SMALT	No	Yes	75
Davido et al (2017)[33]	8	Prospective, multicenter, open-label, uncontrolled	CRE, VRE	No	No	37.5
Dinh et al (2018)[34]	17	Prospective, multicenter, open-label, uncontrolled	CRE, VRE	No	No	CRE: 50 VRE: 87.5 Overall: 62.5
Saidani et al (2018)[35]	10	Retrospective, single-center, case-control	CRE, CR-ACTB	Oral colistin and AMG for 5 days or oral sulfadiazine and fusidic acid if AMG resistant for 5 days	Yes	80

(continued)

Table 10.5-2 (continued). Fecal Microbiota Transplantation for Antibiotic-Resistant Bacteria Decolonization Without Concomitant *Clostridioides difficile* Infection

Author (Year)	N	Study Design	Target Organisms	Antibiotic as Prep	Multiple FMT	Decolonization %
Singh et al (2018)[36]	15	Prospective, single-center, open-label, uncontrolled	ESBL	No	Yes	40
Huttner et al (2019)[37]	22	Prospective, randomized open-label, unblinded, multicenter superiority trial	ESBL, CRE	Oral colistin and neomycin for 5 days	No	41[a]
Davido et al (2019)[32]	8	Prospective, single-center, open-label, uncontrolled	VRE	No	No	62.5 at 1 month; 87.5 at 3 months
Battipaglia et al (2019)[30]	10	Retrospective cohort	VRE, CRE, CRPA	No	Yes	60

Abbreviations: ACTB = *Acinetobacter*; AMG = aminoglycoside; CRPA = carbapenem resistant *Pseudomonas aeruginosa*; CR-ACTB = carbapenem resistant *Acinetobacter baumannii*; MIU = million international units; SMALT = *Stenotrophomonas maltophilia*.

[a] 41% vs 29% decolonization with placebo, non-statistically significant

References

1. Centers for Disease Control and Prevention. Antibiotic resistance threats in the United States, 2013. Accessed September 29, 2020. https://www.cdc.gov/drugresistance/threat-report-2013/pdf/ar-threats-2013-508.pdf

2. Mauldin PD, Salgado CD, Hansen IS, Durup DT, Bosso JA. Attributable hospital cost and length of stay associated with health care-associated infections caused by antibiotic-resistant gram-negative bacteria. *Antimicrob Agents Chemother.* 2010;54(1):109-115.

3. Tseng WP, Chen YC, Chen SY, Chen SY, Chang SC. Risk for subsequent infection and mortality after hospitalization among patients with multidrug-resistant gram-negative bacteria colonization or infection. *Antimicrob Resist Infect Control.* 2018;7:93.

4. Wittekamp BH, Plantinga NL, Cooper BS, et al. Decontamination strategies and bloodstream infections with antibiotic-resistant microorganisms in ventilated patients: a randomized clinical trial. *JAMA.* 2018;320(20):2087-2098.

5. Oren I, Sprecher H, Finkelstein R, et al. Eradication of carbapenem-resistant *Enterobacteriaceae* gastrointestinal colonization with nonabsorbable oral antibiotic treatment: a prospective controlled trial. *Am J Infect Control.* 2013;41(12):1167-1172.

6. Halaby T, Al Naiemi N, Kluytmans J, van der Palen J, Vandenbroucke-Grauls CM. Emergence of colistin resistance in *Enterobacteriaceae* after the introduction of selective digestive tract decontamination in an intensive care unit. *Antimicrob Agents Chemother.* 2013;57(7):3224-3229.

7. Tacconelli E, Mazzaferri F, de Smet AM, et al. ESCMID-EUCIC clinical guidelines on decolonization of multidrug-resistant gram-negative bacteria carriers. *Clin Microbiol Infect.* 2019;25(7):807-817.

8. Lübbert C, Faucheux S, Becker-Rux D, et al. Rapid emergence of secondary resistance to gentamicin and colistin following selective digestive decontamination in patients with KPC-2-producing *Klebsiella pneumoniae*: a single-centre experience. *Int J Antimicrob Agents.* 2013;42(6):565-570.

9. Huttner B, Haustein T, Uçkay I, et al. Decolonization of intestinal carriage of extended-spectrum β-lactamase-producing *Enterobacteriaceae* with oral colistin and neomycin: a randomized, double-blind, placebo-controlled trial. *J Antimicrob Chemother.* 2013;68(10):2375-2382.

10. Millan B, Park H, Hotte N, et al. Fecal microbial transplants reduce antibiotic-resistant genes in patients with recurrent *Clostridium difficile* infection. *Clin Infect Dis.* 2016;62(12):1479-1486.

11. Crum-Cianflone NF, Sullivan E, Ballon-Landa G. Fecal microbiota transplantation and successful resolution of multidrug-resistant-organism colonization. *J Clin Microbiol.* 2015;53(6):1986-1989.

12. Stripling J, Kumar R, Baddley JW, et al. Loss of vancomycin-resistant *Enterococcus* fecal dominance in an organ transplant patient with *Clostridium difficile* colitis after fecal microbiota transplant. *Open Forum Infect Dis.* 2015;2(2):ofv078.

13. Jang MO, An JH, Jung SI, Park KH. Refractory *Clostridium difficile* infection cured with fecal microbiota transplantation in vancomycin-resistant *Enterococcus* colonized patient. *Intest Res.* 2015;13(1):80-84.

14. García-Fernández S, Morosini MI, Cobo M, et al. Gut eradication of VIM-1 producing ST9 Klebsiella oxytoca after fecal microbiota transplantation for diarrhea caused by a *Clostridium difficile* hypervirulent R027 strain. *Diagn Microbiol Infect Dis.* 2016;86(4):470-471.

15. Dubberke ER, Mullane KM, Gerding DN, et al. Clearance of vancomycin-resistant *Enterococcus* concomitant with administration of a microbiota-based drug targeted at recurrent *Clostridium difficile* infection. *Open Forum Infect Dis.* 2016;3(3):ofw133.

16. Santiago M, Eysenbach L, Allegretti J, et al. Microbiome predictors of dysbiosis and VRE decolonization in patients with recurrent *C. difficile* infections in a multi-center retrospective study. *AIMS Microbiol.* 2019;5(1):1-18. doi: 10.3934/microbiol.2019.1.1

17. Sohn KM, Cheon S, Kim YS. Can fecal microbiota transplantation (FMT) eradicate fecal colonization with vancomycin-resistant *Enterococci* (VRE)? *Infect Control Hosp Epidemiol.* 2016;37(12):1519-1521. doi: 10.1017/ice.2016.229

18. Innes AJ, Mullish BH, Fernando F, et al. Faecal microbiota transplant: a novel biological approach to extensively drug-resistant organism-related non-relapse mortality. *Bone Marrow Transplant.* 2017;52(10):1452-1454.

19. Tariq R, Pardi DS, Tosh PK, Walker RC, Razonable RR, Khanna S. Fecal microbiota transplantation for recurrent *Clostridium difficile* infection reduces recurrent urinary tract infection frequency. *Clin Infect Dis.* 2017;65(10):1745-1747.

20. Ponte A, Pinho R, Mota M. Fecal microbiota transplantation: is there a role in the eradication of carbapenem-resistant *Klebsiella pneumoniae* intestinal carriage? *Rev Esp Enferm Dig.* 2017;109(5):392.

21. Wang T, Kraft CS, Woodworth MH, Dhere T, Eaton ME. Fecal microbiota transplant for refractory *Clostridium difficile* infection interrupts 25-year history of recurrent urinary tract infections. *Open Forum Infect Dis.* 2018;5(2):ofy016.

22. Santiago M, Eysenbach L, Allegretti J, et al. Microbiome predictors of dysbiosis and VRE decolonization in patients with recurrent *C. difficile* infections in a multi-center retrospective study. *AIMS Microbiol.* 2019;5(1):1-18.

23. Özsoy S, İlki A. Detection of vancomycin-resistant enterococci (VRE) in stool specimens submitted for *Clostridium difficile* toxin testing. *Braz J Microbiol.* 2017;48(3):489-492.

24. Biliński J, Grzesiowski P, Muszyński J, et al. Fecal microbiota transplantation inhibits multidrug-resistant gut pathogens: preliminary report performed in an immunocompromised host. *Arch Immunol Ther Exp (Warsaw).* 2016;64(3):255-258.

25. Freedman A, Eppes S. Use of stool transplant to clear fecal colonization with carbapenem-resistant *Enterobacteraciae* (CRE): proof of concept. *Open Forum Infect Dis.* 2014;1(suppl 1):S65.

26. Lahtinen P, Mattila E, Anttila VJ, et al. Faecal microbiota transplantation in patients with *Clostridium difficile* and significant comorbidities as well as in patients with new indications: a case series. *World J Gastroenterol.* 2017;23(39):7174-7184.

27. Lagier JC, Million M, Fournier PE, Brouqui P, Raoult D. Faecal microbiota transplantation for stool decolonization of OXA-48 carbapenemase-producing *Klebsiella pneumoniae. J Hosp Infect.* 2015;90(2):173-174.

28. Singh R, van Nood E, Nieuwdorp M, et al. Donor feces infusion for eradication of extended spectrum beta-lactamase producing *Escherichia coli* in a patient with end stage renal disease. *Clin Microbiol Infect.* 2014;20(11):O977-O978.

29. Stalenhoef JE, Terveer EM, Knetsch CW, et al. Fecal microbiota transfer for multidrug-resistant gram-negatives: a clinical success combined with microbiological failure. *Open Forum Infect Dis.* 2017;4(2):ofx047.

30. Battipaglia G, Malard F, Rubio MT, et al. Fecal microbiota transplantation before or after allogeneic hematopoietic transplantation in patients with hematologic malignancies carrying multidrug-resistance bacteria. *Haematologica.* 2019;104(8):1682-1688.

31. Biliński J, Grzesiowski P, Sorensen N, et al. Fecal microbiota transplantation in patients with blood disorders inhibits gut colonization with antibiotic-resistant bacteria: results of a prospective, single-center study. *Clin Infect Dis.* 2017;65(3):364-370.

32. Davido B, Batista R, Fessi H, et al. Fecal microbiota transplantation to eradicate vancomycin-resistant enterococci colonization in case of an outbreak. *Med Mal Infect.* 2019;49(3):214-218.

33. Davido B, Batista R, Michelon H, et al. Is faecal microbiota transplantation an option to eradicate highly drug-resistant enteric bacteria carriage? *J Hosp Infect.* 2017;95(4):433-437.

34. Dinh A, Fessi H, Duran C, et al. Clearance of carbapenem-resistant *Enterobacteriaceae* vs vancomycin-resistant *Enterococci* carriage after faecal microbiota transplant: a prospective comparative study. *J Hosp Infect.* 2018;99(4):481-486.

35. Saïdani N, Lagier JC, Cassir N, et al. Faecal microbiota transplantation shortens the colonisation period and allows re-entry of patients carrying carbapenamase-producing bacteria into medical care facilities. *Int J Antimicrob Agents.* 2019;53(4):355-361.

36. Singh R, de Groot PF, Geerlings SE, et al. Fecal microbiota transplantation against intestinal colonization by extended spectrum beta-lactamase producing Enterobacteriaceae: a proof of principle study. *BMC Res Notes.* 2018;11(1):190.

37. Huttner BD, de Lastours V, Wassenberg M, et al. A 5-day course of oral antibiotics followed by faecal transplantation to eradicate carriage of multidrug-resistant Enterobacteriaceae: a randomized clinical trial. *Clin Microbiol Infect.* 2019;25(7):830-838.

38. Wei Y, Gong J, Zhu W, et al. Fecal microbiota transplantation restores dysbiosis in patients with methicillin resistant *Staphylococcus aureus* enterocolitis. *BMC Infect Dis.* 2015;15:265. doi: 10.1186/s12879-015-0973-1

10.6

The Role of Fecal Microbiota Transplantation in the Treatment of Obesity, Metabolic Syndrome, and Nonalcoholic Fatty Liver Disease

Benjamin H. Mullish, MB, BChir, MRCP, PhD

Over the course of the past decade, there has been a growing literature base of observational studies demonstrating an association between the interrelated metabolic conditions of obesity, metabolic syndrome, and NAFLD and alterations in the composition and functionality of the gut microbiota. Animal models and emerging human studies have begun to explore this association mechanistically. The success of FMT in treating rCDI has been a launch pad for interest in its potential application in metabolic conditions where perturbation of the gut microbiota may contribute to the pathology observed and where current medical therapy may be limited. In this section, we will summarize the current knowledge within this area.

Allegretti JR, Kassam Z, eds. *The 6 Ds of Fecal Microbiota Transplantation: A Primer From Decision to Discharge and Beyond* (pp 169-175).
© 2021 SLACK Incorporated.

Overview of the Role of the Gut Microbiota in Obesity, Metabolic Syndrome, and Nonalcoholic Fatty Liver Disease

Multiple cross-sectional studies have demonstrated that individuals with obesity have alterations in their gut microbiota,[1] and individuals with a gut microbiota of low bacterial richness have more marked insulin resistance and dyslipidemia compared with those with a higher bacterial richness.[2] In addition, women with normal, impaired, or diabetic glucose control were able to be identified based upon the composition and functionality of their stool microbiome profile.[3]

A range of animal models, including humanized mouse models, have demonstrated that vulnerability to obesity and metabolic syndrome may be transferred with transfer of the gut microbiota, giving further circumstantial evidence for the contribution of the gut microbiota to these conditions. This includes studies in which stool from human twins discordant for obesity has been transferred into the gut of germ-free mice (ie, mice lacking a microbiota), with mice receiving stool from the obese twin gaining much more weight than those treated with stool from the nonobese twin.[4] Furthermore, there is evidence from animal models that the metabolic improvements observed post-bariatric surgery may be causally related to surgery-related changes in the gut microbiota.[5] One prominent theory is that the obese gut microbiota has an increased capacity to harvest energy from the host's diet, with the major consequence being fat deposition and its associated sequelae.[6]

Using a combination of samples collected from patients with morbid obesity and mouse models, it has recently been demonstrated that the microbial metabolite phenylacetic acid may be contributory to the development of hepatic steatosis, and, by extension, to the development and progression of NAFLD.[7]

One possible mechanistic explanation for the association between alterations in the gut microbiota and vulnerability to and development of these conditions includes alterations in the level of production of gut bacterial fermentation products, such as short-chain fatty acids (SCFAs). SCFAs appear to mediate the release of the gut peptide glucagon-like peptide-1 (GLP-1), which has actions including the promotion of satiety and slowing of gastric emptying, among others. The gut microbiota also influences the composition of the gut bile acid pool, which in turn may directly impact upon host lipid metabolism and weight.[8,9]

Clinical Trials of Fecal Microbiota Transplantation for Treating Obesity, Metabolic Syndrome, and Nonalcoholic Fatty Liver Disease

A high-profile case report from 2015 described rapid, marked weight gain in a woman who was treated for rCDI with FMT obtained from her healthy but overweight daughter,[10] raising interest in the possible direct transferability of obesity as a gut microbiota trait in humans. However, larger studies have failed to replicate this observation, and it is now widely accepted that stool donor body mass index (BMI) does not appear to affect recipient weight after FMT for rCDI.[11]

In 2 randomized studies reported from the same academic group, collectively including 56 white, male, obese, treatment-naïve patients with metabolic syndrome, a significant improvement was demonstrated in peripheral (but not hepatic) insulin sensitivity following 1 to 2 upper GI infusions of lean donor FMT.[12,13] This improvement was observed at 6 weeks post-FMT but was no longer present at later time points. However, no improvement in insulin sensitivity occurred in patients treated with autologous FMT (ie, patients transplanted with their own collected feces).[12,13] Importantly, these findings were observed without the use of maintenance FMT, raising the possibility that with an increased dosing schedule, improvements in insulin sensitivity may have been sustained. Of note, lean donor FMT was not associated with changes in weight or other relevant metabolic parameters. The effect of FMT upon the levels of fecal SCFAs was variable between patients, but relatively modest overall.

Allegretti et al[14] conducted a randomized clinical trial where 22 patients with obesity (BMI ≥ 35 kg/m^2) but without other metabolic diseases (ie, no NAFLD, diabetes mellitus, or other features of metabolic syndrome) were randomized to receive either FMT or placebo (Figure 10.6-1).[14] FMT was administered as capsules derived from a single lean donor (BMI 17.5 kg/m^2) divided over 3 doses (30 capsules at induction and 12 capsules at week 4 and week 8). Although FMT appeared overall safe and well-tolerated, no significant changes in GLP-1, the primary endpoint, or in BMI were seen across 12 weeks of follow-up. It was further observed that patients who received FMT, but not those who received placebo, demonstrated particular changes in the microbiome and bile acid profiles of the gut to resemble that of donors. In another randomized placebo-controlled trial, 24 obese adults with mild-to-moderate insulin resistance were randomized to receive 6 weekly

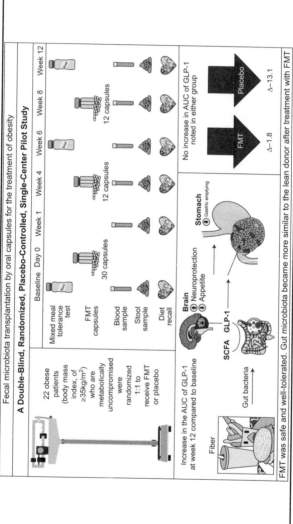

Figure 10.6-1. Fecal microbiota transplantation by oral capsules for the treatment of obesity.[14]

treatments with capsules of either a metabolically healthy lean donor FMT or placebo and were followed for up to 12 weeks.[15] Although there were numerically greater improvements in insulin sensitivity in the FMT group compared with the placebo arm, this did not reach statistical significance.[15]

In an additional study, 22 patients with metabolic syndrome were given FMT from either a donor with metabolic syndrome or a donor who had undergone bariatric surgery (via Roux-en-Y gastric bypass [RYGB]).[16] Patients receiving FMT from donors with metabolic syndrome experienced a marked reduction in peripheral insulin sensitivity at 2 weeks post-FMT, while this was not seen in those receiving FMT from donors post-RYGB.[16]

At present, only one randomized trial has been published investigating the impact of FMT in patients with NAFLD,[17] although several more are being undertaken, and other early studies have presented preliminary data. The published randomized trial, which included 21 participants, observed that small intestinal permeability was significantly improved at 6 weeks post-FMT in patients with increased gut leak at baseline who received healthy donor FMT, but not in those receiving autologous FMT.[17] However, no FMT-related improvements in other relevant clinical parameters (including insulin resistance or hepatic fat) were observed. Data from a further pilot study in which lean donor FMT was administered to the upper GI tract of patients with NASH but without cirrhosis showed that FMT appeared to be safe overall in these groups; however, no improvement in liver fat was detected at 12 weeks post-FMT in the 3 patients completing the protocol.[18] For further discussion, see Chapter 10.3: "The Role of Fecal Microbiota Transplantation in the Treatment of Liver Diseases."

Summary

Results to date regarding FMT as a possible treatment for obesity, metabolic syndrome, and NAFLD have been mixed. On one hand, studies have tended to demonstrate restoration of gut microbiota composition (and sometimes functionality) to resemble that of the donor, and a transient improvement in insulin resistance may occur. Conversely, no sustained improvement in any metrics of clinical significance has been observed, although studies rarely use maintenance FMT.

Within this field, there is already interest in potentially moving beyond FMT to more targeted microbiome therapies. For examples, there is a reported negative correlation between the abundance of the bacterium *Akkermansia muciniphila* within the gut and clinical features of the metabolic syndrome[19]; as such, a recent double-blind, placebo-controlled randomized trial administered either *A. muciniphila* (10^{10} colony-forming units, either live or pasteurized) or placebo as an oral treatment daily for 3 months to 32 patients who were overweight/obese with insulin resistance.[20] Patients receiving *A. muciniphila* experienced significantly improved insulin sensitivity and plasma total cholesterol compared with those receiving placebo, as well as trends toward improvement in other metabolic parameters.[20] A range of different comparable clinical studies are at varying stages of planning and recruitment.

Overall, there is a great deal of future work to perform in this area. For instance, as a growing understanding of the mechanistic contribution of the gut microbiota to obesity develops, so future clinical FMT studies in this area may allow more nuanced donor selection (eg, on the basis of particular enrichment of specific microbiota functionalities).[21] A further added complexity is that the gut microbiota appears to at least partly mediate the clinical effects of certain medications used commonly in these patient groups, including antidiabetic medications, such as metformin,[22] which may also influence trial design.

References

1. Ley RE, Bäckhed F, Turnbaugh P, Lozupone CA, Knight RD, Gordon JI. Obesity alters gut microbial ecology. *Proc Natl Acad Sci U S A*. 2005;102(31):11070-11075.

2. Le Chatelier E, Nielsen T, Qin J, et al. Richness of human gut microbiome correlates with metabolic markers. *Nature*. 2013;500(7464):541-546.

3. Karlsson FH, Tremaroli V, Nookaew I, et al. Gut metagenome in European women with normal, impaired and diabetic glucose control. *Nature*. 2013;498(7452):99-103.

4. Ridaura VK, Faith JJ, Rey FE, et al. Gut microbiota from twins discordant for obesity modulate metabolism in mice. *Science*. 2013;341(6150):1241214.

5. Liou AP, Paziuk M, Luevano JM Jr, Machineni S, Turnbaugh PJ, Kaplan LM. Conserved shifts in the gut microbiota due to gastric bypass reduce host weight and adiposity. *Sci Transl Med*. 2013;5(178):178ra41.

6. Turnbaugh PJ, Ley RE, Mahowald MA, Magrini V, Mardis ER, Gordon JI. An obesity-associated gut microbiome with increased capacity for energy harvest. *Nature*. 2006;444(7122):1027-1031.

7. Hoyles L, Fernández-Real JM, Federici M, et al. Molecular phenomics and metagenomics of hepatic steatosis in non-diabetic obese women. *Nat Med*. 2018;24(7):1070-1080.

8. Joyce SA, MacSharry J, Casey PG, et al. Regulation of host weight gain and lipid metabolism by bacterial bile acid modification in the gut. *Proc Natl Acad Sci U S A*. 2014;111(20):7421-7426.

9. Cani PD, Van Hul M, Lefort C, Depommier C, Rastelli M, Everard A. Microbial regulation of organismal energy homeostasis. *Nat Metab*. 2019;1(1):34-46.

10. Alang N, Kelly CR. Weight gain after fecal microbiota transplantation. *Open Forum Infect Dis*. 2015;2(1):ofv004.

11. Fischer M, Kao D, Kassam Z, et al. Stool donor body mass index does not affect recipient weight after a single fecal microbiota transplantation for *Clostridium difficile* infection. *Clin Gastroenterol Hepatol.* 2018;16(8):1351-1353.

12. Vrieze A, Van Nood E, Holleman F, et al. Transfer of intestinal microbiota from lean donors increases insulin sensitivity in individuals with metabolic syndrome. *Gastroenterology.* 2012;143(4):913-916.e7.

13. Kootte RS, Levin E, Salojärvi J, et al. Improvement of insulin sensitivity after lean donor feces in metabolic syndrome is driven by baseline intestinal microbiota composition. *Cell Metab.* 2017;26(4):611-619.e6.

14. Allegretti JR, Kassam Z, Mullish BH, et al. Effects of fecal microbiota transplantation with oral capsules in obese patients. *Clin Gastroenterol Hepatol.* 2020;18(4):855-863.e2.

15. Yu EW, Gao L, Stastka P, et al. Fecal microbiota transplantation for the improvement of metabolism in obesity: The FMT-TRIM double-blind placebo-controlled pilot trial. *PLoS Med.* 2020;17(3):e1003051.

16. de Groot P, Scheithauer T, Bakker GJ, et al. Donor metabolic characteristics drive effects of faecal microbiota transplantation on recipient insulin sensitivity, energy expenditure and intestinal transit time. *Gut.* 2020;69(3):502-512.

17. Craven L, Rahman A, Parvathy SN, et al. Allogenic fecal microbiota transplantation in patients with nonalcoholic fatty liver disease improves abnormal small intestinal permeability: a randomized clinical trial. *Am J Gastroenterol.* 2020;115(7):1055-1065. doi: 10.14309/ajg.0000000000000661

18. Wungjiranirun M, Risech-Neyman Y, Wang C, Grand DJ, Kelly CR, Promrat K. Fecal microbiota transplantation in nonalcoholic steatohepatitis: a case series. *Gastroenterology.* 2019;156(6 suppl 1):S1237.

19. Cani PD, Van Hul M, Lefort C, Depommier C, Rastelli M, Everard A. Microbial regulation of organismal energy homeostasis. *Nat Metab.* 2019;1(1):34-46.

20. Depommier C, Everard A, Druart C, et al. Supplementation with *Akkermansia muciniphila* in overweight and obese human volunteers: a proof-of-concept exploratory study. *Nat Med.* 2019;25(7):1096-1103.

21. Allegretti JR, Mullish BH, Kelly C, Fischer M. The evolution of the use of faecal microbiota transplantation and emerging therapeutic indications. *Lancet.* 2019;394(10196):420-431.

22. Sun L, Xie C, Wang G, et al. Gut microbiota and intestinal FXR mediate the clinical benefits of metformin. *Nat Med.* 2018;24(12):1919-1929.

11

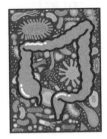

Frequently Asked Questions

Jessica R. Allegretti, MD, MPH and
Zain Kassam, MD, MPH

Given that the field of fecal microbiota transplantation (FMT) and microbiome therapeutics is relatively new, there are many questions that arise from both patients and providers for its use in *Clostridioides difficile* infection (CDI) and beyond. This chapter provides a practical reference to frequently asked questions (FAQs) that patients ask FMT clinicians and frequent inquiries from clinicians when first starting to treat patients with FMT.

Allegretti JR, Kassam Z, eds. *The 6 Ds of Fecal Microbiota Transplantation: A Primer From Decision to Discharge and Beyond* (pp 177-190).
© 2021 SLACK Incorporated.

Patient FAQs: Common Questions From Patients Referred to You for Fecal Microbiota Transplantation

This sounds experimental. Why should I have this procedure done?

- With each episode of CDI, the risk of a recurrence becomes exponentially more likely. Once a patient has 3 or more confirmed episodes of CDI, it is unlikely that additional courses of *C. difficile* antibiotics (eg, vancomycin, fidaxomicin) alone will lead to a sustained clinical cure. Additional antibiotics alone are likely to result in ongoing disruption of the patient's intestinal microbiome.

- FMT is still considered investigational therapy by the US Food and Drug Administration (FDA); however, its use is recommended in both US and European clinical practice guidelines for the prevention of recurrent CDI (rCDI) following standard-of-care (SOC) *C. difficile* antibiotics.

- Overall, FMT appears well-tolerated, and current data suggest the short-term safety profile is favorable as long as there is robust donor screening. Long-term data are still emerging; however, the current data suggest FMT does not have a concerning long-term safety profile (see Chapter 7: "Discussion: How Do You Discuss the Risks and Benefits of Fecal Microbiota Transplantation?").

- The majority of patients with rCDI will be cured after a single FMT following SOC *C. difficile* antibiotics.

If I have a fecal microbiota transplantation, does this mean I will never get Clostridioides difficile infection again?

- Unfortunately, you cannot guarantee your patient will never get CDI again. FMT is used to reduce the risk of subsequent CDI episodes and break the cycle of recurrence they are currently in.

- There is always the possibility of CDI in the future, especially in the setting of systemic antibiotic use. CDI patients who undergo an FMT and have no recurrence at 8 weeks post-intervention have an approximately 10% chance of having another CDI episode, and this risk is mainly derived from future courses of antibiotics. Patients who have systemic antibiotic exposure after FMT but prior to week 8 have an approximately 3-fold risk of CDI recurrence compared with those who do not receive antibiotics.

Do I have to provide my own donor?

- We recommend you follow institutional best practices regarding procuring material from a patient-selected or universal donor. Most commonly, health care facilities use the universal donor approach, leveraging banked material either from an external stool bank or from a hospital-based stool bank. Patient-selected donors who complete the same screening procedures can be used, although there can be operational challenges. In some rare clinical situations, patient-selected donors may be the recommended donor strategy (see Chapter 6: "Donor: How Do You Select and Screen Candidate Donors for Fecal Microbiota Transplantation?").

How long do I have to retain the material after the fecal microbiota transplantation?

- Retention of material after lower gastrointestinal (GI) administration (eg, colonoscopy, flexible sigmoidoscopy, enema) can often be difficult, especially in older patients with poor baseline sphincter control. There are limited data to suggest that longer retention leads to better outcomes.

- We recommend the patients retain the material while they are in the procedure recovery unit. However, if this is not possible, it is important to counsel patients that it is not an issue if they are unable to retain and it is not likely to impact the results. Given that the material is often infused into the right colon or cecum, the first material the patients will pass is likely their own residual stool and bowel preparation because no suctioning is done on the withdrawal of the endoscope.

- It is reasonable to have patients use the restroom before they leave the endoscopy unit, especially for those with long commutes.

- It is recommended to offer patients an absorbent pad/undergarment to ensure no leakage on the way home.

- The administration of loperamide prior to the FMT can be considered to assist with retention; however, there are no data to suggest this will improve outcomes, and most experts do not use loperamide.

When will I know if the fecal microbiota transplantation worked?

- Most patients will describe feeling better within 24 hours of the FMT procedure.
- It is common for patients not to have any bowel movements for the first few days post-FMT. This may lead to concern in some patients, so we recommend counseling about this post-FMT constipation phenomenon.
- Clinical cure is generally defined as an absence of CDI through week 8. Approximately 86% of patients who experience a CDI recurrence will do so by week 4, and the mean time to CDI recurrence is approximately 14 days after FMT. Accordingly, you can often provide reassurance to your patients that there is a high likelihood of clinical cure if they have not experienced a CDI recurrence by week 4 post-FMT.

Am going to taste or smell poop?

- No! This is a common misconception. Patients who undergo an FMT via colonoscopy will eventually pass the material that is indistinguishable from their own stool. Anecdotally, patients have reported noticing a different odor to their gas post-FMT.
- Capsule formulations are frozen and have no odor or taste when swallowed. Newer microbiome therapeutic formulations are lyophilized or freeze-dried capsules that are shelf-stable, have no odor or taste, and eliminate any indication that the material was derived from human stool.

Am I going to get fat?

- There has been a single high-publicity case report of weight gain after FMT from a donor who is overweight. Importantly, a large cohort study (N = 173) refuted the case report's finding and suggested that a stool donor's body mass index did not affect a recipient's weight after a single FMT for CDI. Regardless, out of an abundance of caution, donors must be normal weight, and therefore it is unlikely for patients who receive FMT to become obese.
- It is important to counsel patient about healthy weight gain post-FMT. Most patients lose weight during their CDI course; therefore, a healthy weight regain is expected. This has been shown to not exceed their pre-CDI baseline.

Would you recommend at-home fecal microbiota transplantation?

- No. Using unscreened material at home via a do-it-yourself (DIY) FMT can be dangerous and may lead to transmission of an infection or a microbiome-mediated condition. We would always recommend consultation with a physician and the use of well-screened donor material that is compliant with manufacturing and quality best practices.
- Additionally, many patients interested in DIY FMT are using them to treat diseases other than CDI, and this is not recommended.

Can I do fecal microbiota transplantation if I don't have Clostridioides difficile *infection*?

- FMT is currently only recommended for patients with recurrent or refractory CDI following SOC antibiotics for CDI (see Chapter 4: "Decision: Which Patients with *Clostridioides difficile* Infection Are Appropriate for Fecal Microbiota Transplantation?").
- There are many ongoing clinical trials exploring the use of FMT for other indications. If patients are interested, refer them to www.clinicaltrials.gov or an equivalent trial website to look for clinical trials in your area (see Chapter 10 "Discovery: Emerging Indications").

I don't want to take antibiotics. Can I start with fecal microbiota transplantation to treat my Clostridioides difficile *infection*?

- FMT is only recommended for recurrent or refractory CDI following SOC antibiotics for CDI (see Chapter 4: "Decision: Which Patients With *Clostridioides difficile* Infection Are Appropriate for Fecal Microbiota Transplantation?").
- At this time, FMT is not indicated for a first episode of CDI or primary CDI. We would recommend counseling your patients that approximately 80% of patients will have a clinical cure without further recurrence with an initial treatment course of antibiotics.

Do I need to be on a special diet after my fecal microbiota transplantation?

- No. There are no data to suggest that a specific diet will improve the efficacy the FMT or improve engraftment profiles. The most important consideration post-FMT is limiting the use of unnecessary systemic antibiotics.

Can the transplant reject?

- This procedure, although referred to as a transplant, does not carry the same requirements for organ matching that is conducted in solid organ transplantation (SOT), and traditional immunological rejection is not a concern.
- Engraftment is used to determine whether the FMT took. Engraftment generally means that microbes were absent in the patient pre-FMT, found in the donor, and detected in the patient after FMT.
- Engraftment is not used in clinical practice. Instead, clinical cure is used to determine the success of FMT among patients with CDI.

Provider FAQs:
Common Questions From Clinicians Considering Performing a Fecal Microbiota Transplantation or Referring a Patient for a Fecal Microbiota Transplantation

Should patients be banking their own stool for later use?

- Currently, this process is generally not done in clinical practice. However, there has been preliminary proof-of-concept work in self-banking, and there may be future utility to a process similar to that of banking cord blood.

Is it safe to do colonoscopy in patients with Clostridioides difficile *infection?*

- Yes! This procedure is meant to be performed for the prevention of CDI recurrence. Accordingly, patients will be on SOC *C. difficile* antibiotics, followed by an FMT. The colons of rCDI patients are generally not inflamed and usually appear endoscopically normal on luminal visualization.

- Procedurally, no special considerations are required during FMT; however, you may consider using carbon dioxide instead of oxygen for insufflation because there will be minimal or no suctioning upon the withdrawal of the endoscope.

- Standard infection control measures should be implemented in the endoscopy unit

Is bowel preparation required prior to fecal microbiota transplantation?

- Although there is speculation on the role of bowel preparation on decreasing residual *C. difficile* spores in the colon and/or removing residual *C. difficile* antibiotics (eg, vancomycin), there are limited data on the use of standard bowel preparation prior to FMT regardless of delivery modality.

- Bowel preparation is recommended prior to FMT via colonoscopy for luminal visualization and ruling out colonic pathology that may mimic clinical CDI (eg, microscopic colitis, ulcerative colitis, Crohn's disease).

- Generally, bowel preparation is not administered prior to upper GI administration (eg, nasogastric tube [NGT]) or FMT capsules.

How do I refer a patient for a fecal microbiota transplantation if I'm not comfortable doing it myself?

- Stool banks often have a provider list of health care facilities they supply.

- National gastroenterology or infectious disease medical societies may also have clinician contacts for FMT or ongoing national FMT registries. For example, the American Gastroenterological Association has sponsored the US FMT Registry, and a list of all participating sites appears on www.clinicaltrials.gov

If the fecal microbiota transplantation doesn't work, what should I do next?

- In the context of suspected FMT failure, it is important to confirm that the diagnosis of rCDI and to rule out mimics such as post-infection irritable bowel syndrome with *C. difficile* colonization (see Chapter 4: "Decision: Which Patients With *Clostridioides difficile* Infection Are Appropriate for Fecal Microbiota Transplantation?").

- Clinically, there are several factors that increase the risk for FMT failure. These include severe or fulminant CDI at the time of FMT, the presence of pseudomembranes, ongoing use of systemic antibiotics post-FMT, and certain comorbidities or immunocompromised states, including SOT and inflammatory bowel disease (IBD). Counseling patients about the risk of FMT failure must be done during the informed consent process (see Chapter 7: "Discussion: How Do You Discuss the Risks and Benefits of Fecal Microbiota Transplantation?").

- There are generally 3 categories of FMT failure:
  1. Primary nonresponse: This is defined as ongoing diarrhea with laboratory-confirmed *C. difficile* testing immediately after or within 7 days of the FMT. The patient never experiences sustained relief. In this case, it is appropriate to start an abbreviated course of SOC *C. difficile* antibiotics and bring the patient back quickly for a repeat FMT (typically 1 week later).

  2. Secondary nonresponse: This is defined as a patient who experiences resolution of his or her diarrhea after FMT; however, the diarrhea returns with laboratory-confirmed *C. difficile* testing between 1 and 8 weeks after the FMT. Early secondary nonresponse is between weeks 1 and 4, and late secondary nonresponse is between weeks 4 and 8. It is important to confirm CDI recurrence with a 2-stage testing algorithm (see Chapter 4: "Decision: Which Patients With *Clostridioides difficile* Infection Are Appropriate for Fecal Microbiota Transplantation?"). If CDI recurrence is confirmed, it is appropriate to repeat FMT. It is appropriate to restart vancomycin for a minimum of 4 days to help improve symptoms and reduce colonic inflammation prior to FMT, although longer courses are also reasonable.

  3. Reinfection: If the patient experiences a CDI recurrence after 8 weeks post-FMT, this should be considered a new primary CDI episode. Repeat FMT does not need to be performed, and treatment with SOC *C. difficile* antibiotics is appropriate.

- Overall, data suggest that FMT failure rates are higher with naso-enteric administration and enema. Therefore, if your patients experience FMT failure after FMT, you should consider administration with colonoscopy or high-efficacy FMT capsules.

- Some experts suggest FMT administration into both the jejunum and colon by combined push enteroscopy and colonoscopy for patients with multiple confirmed FMT failures.

Should I test my patient for cure after the fecal microbiota transplantation? What test should I be using?

- No, testing for cure post-FMT is not required. In the absence of CDI symptoms, repeat *C. difficile* laboratory testing to assess to confirm cure or to assess for ongoing colonization is not needed. In fact, >95% of patients will be decolonized after a successful FMT.

- Should persistent diarrhea (Bristol stool score [BSS] 6-7) return and there is clinical suspicion for CDI, laboratory testing should be done to confirm CDI recurrence. If testing is negative in the setting of diarrhea, alternative diagnoses should be explored (see Chapter 9: "Discharge: How Should You Follow and Care for Patients After Fecal Microbiota Transplantation?").

Does a patient have to fail a vancomycin taper in order to qualify for a fecal microbiota transplantation?

- No. Indication for FMT is determined by the number of confirmed episodes of CDI or disease severity, not by prior treatment courses (see Chapter 4: "Decision: Which Patients With *Clostridioides difficile* Infection Are Appropriate for Fecal Microbiota Transplantation?").

Is it safe to do biopsies or take out polyps during fecal microbiota transplantation?

- Yes. If there is any concern about potential other causes of the patient's diarrhea that need to be explored (eg, microscopic colitis or IBD), obtaining random or targeted biopsies at the time of FMT is appropriate.

- Most experts believe that removing polyps is generally safe at the time of FMT.

- It is important to counsel patients that FMT via colonoscopy does not count as a standard screening colonoscopy. Visualization of the lumen is obscured upon the withdrawal of the scope due to administration of the donor material. If you feel that a screening colonoscopy must be done at the time of FMT, you will need to perform a full colonoscopy with appropriate withdrawal and inspection and then reenter the colon to deliver the material, preferably in the cecum. If this is not possible or you do not feel comfortable, the patient should come back at a later date to have a full screening colonoscopy.

How fast do you infuse the fecal microbiota transplantation material?

- In endoscopic administration (eg, upper endoscopy, colonoscopy, flexible sigmoidoscopy), there is no preferred speed of infusion. The material can either be drawn up into 60-cc syringes and manually pushed through the biopsy cap, similar to a water flush, or the bottle can be hooked up to the water foot pedal and pumped through the endoscope.

- In enema administration, the 250 mL of material can be transferred to an enema bag and infused over 1 hour to patients in the left lateral decubitus position. Patients should attempt retention of the material for 1 hour, although there is a paucity of data on the timing. Preferably, patients should be asked to periodically rotate 180 degrees to the right side and back to help distribute the material throughout the colon. However, if the patient has mobility issues, the rotation step may be omitted from the procedure.

- In NGT administration, patients should be positioned upright during administration. Smaller-volume material is used in the upper GI tract (see Chapter 8: "Delivery: How Do You Select the Most Appropriate Delivery Modality for Fecal Microbiota Transplantation?"). Material can be infused over 2 to 3 minutes. Once complete, the NGT can be removed 30 minutes after the infusion is complete, and patients should remain upright to reduce risk of aspiration. Patients should be observed post-procedure for between 30 minutes and 2 hours to ensure no aspiration-related adverse events.

For fulminant Clostridioides difficile infection patients, is it safe to do a flexible sigmoidoscopy at the bedside? Am I going to cause a perforation?

- Unlike patients with rCDI, fulminant CDI patients will have acutely inflamed colons. However, gentle flexible sigmoidoscopy by a skilled endoscopist can still be safely performed. The aim is to assess the colon for pseudomembranes and deliver the material to the most proximal part of the colon that can be reached safely. Carbon dioxide is highly recommended in these patients to minimize distention, and light insufflation should be employed.

- An upper endoscope can be used for the procedure; gentle insertion and direct visualization is recommended.

- Enema administration in this population has been considered. A drawback to enema administration in fulminant CDI patients is the lack of direct visualization to assess for pseudomembranes, which is often needed for sequential FMT protocols (see Chapter 10.1.2: "The Role of Fecal Microbiota Transplantation in the Treatment of Severe and Fulminant *Clostridioides difficile* Infection"). Additionally, lower efficacy has been reported with enema in fulminant patients. If performing multiple flexible sigmoidoscopies is not feasible, you can consider administering of the first FMT via flexible sigmoidoscopy and subsequent FMTs via enema.

How does fecal microbiota transplantation work?

- The mechanism of FMT for the prevention of rCDI has not been fully elucidated; however, there are 2 primary hypotheses linked to the restoration of the gut microbiome. First, patients with rCDI have a lower microbiome diversity than healthy individuals or those with primary CDI. A high-diversity environment restored by FMT is thought to provide colonization resistance and prevent *C. difficile* from colonizing and subsequently producing toxin. Second, patients with rCDI have a decrease in secondary bile acids compared with healthy individuals or those with primary CDI. This is thought to be due to disruption of the healthy gut microbiome, which impacts bile acid ratios (primary vs secondary bile acids). Secondary bile acids prevent *C. difficile* spores from transforming into an active vegetative state capable of producing toxin. FMT helps restore a healthy gut microbiome, and in turn restore a healthy bile acid profile.

Do you have to match donors?

- This procedure, although referred to as a transplant, does not carry the same requirements for matching that is done in SOT.

- We do not currently match donors and recipient based on age, gender, or other immune factors, such as human leukocyte antigen matching.

- In fact, the efficacy of FMT for the prevention of CDI recurrence is so high, there are no specific donor factors that have been found that directly correlate with higher efficacy rates. This includes microbiome profiles, donor diet, donor short-chain fatty acid profiles, BSS of donation, and donor stool processing time.

Are we still calling this fecal microbiota transplantation?

- This therapy has several names, including *fecal microbiota transplantation*, *stool transplant*, *stool transfer*, *fecal transplant*, *intestinal microbiota transplant* or *transfer*, and *intestinal microbiome restoration*, among others. These all refer to the same therapeutic intervention.

- Fecal microbiota transplantation, or FMT, is currently the most commonly used term. However, many clinicians feel that it is not patient-centric and that having the term *fecal* or *stool* in the title is not appropriate because the engraftment of intestinal microbiota is the critical component of this procedure. Therefore, *intestinal microbiota transfer* may be more appropriate.

Is there any role for fecal microbiota transplantation in oncology?

- Graft vs host disease (GvHD) in the gut: There are emerging data on the role of the microbiome in hematology-oncology patients who have undergone stem cell transplantations. An international study of 1362 patients undergoing allogeneic hematopoietic cell transplantation demonstrated that these patients were characterized by a loss of microbiome diversity and that high diversity was associated with a lower risk of death.[1] Clinician-scientists have also specifically applied FMT to increase microbiome diversity for GI GvHD, with encouraging preliminary results. A systematic review and meta-analysis of 37 GvHD patients who underwent FMT reported a 74% response rate with a well-tolerated safety profile.[2] Well-designed controlled studies are required, but microbiome diagnostics and therapeutics may have a role in the future care of hematology-oncology patients.

- Combination therapy with immune checkpoint inhibitors (ICIs): Immunotherapy has revolutionized oncology care; however, programmed cell death protein 1/programmed death-ligand 1 and cytotoxic T-lymphocyte–associated protein 4 inhibitors are not effective in all patients. Landmark preclinical data suggest that the gut microbiome plays a key critical role in the efficacy of immunotherapies for cancer.[3] Accordingly, there are ongoing studies that are assessing the role of FMT in combination with ICI in a number of different cancer types, as well as ICI nonresponders.

- ICI colitis: ICI colitis is a common immune-related adverse event associated with ICIs used in oncology. Typically, it occurs after weeks after the second or third dose, and, endoscopically and histologically, the presentation is nearly identical to IBD. Recent reports suggest that FMT may have a role in steroid-refractory cases by reconstituting the microbiome and increasing the proportion of regulatory T-cells in the colonic mucosa.[4] Further research is needed, but FMT remains a promising option for ICI colitis.

References

1. Peled JU, Gomes ALC, Devlin SM, et al. Microbiota as predictor of mortality in allogeneic hematopoietic-cell transplantation. *N Engl J Med*. 2020;382:822-834.
2. Tariq R, Furqan F, Pardi D, Khanna S. Efficacy of fecal microbiota transplantation for acute graft versus host disease in the gut: a systematic review and meta-analysis. *Am J Gastroenterol*. 2019;114:S123.
3. Routy B, Le Chatelier E, Derosa L, et al. Gut microbiome influences efficacy of PD-1–based immunotherapy against epithelial tumors. *Science*. 2018;359:91-97.
4. Wang Y, Wiesnoski DH, Helmink BA, et al. Fecal microbiota transplantation for refractory immune checkpoint inhibitor-associated colitis. *Nat Med*. 2018;24(12):1804-1808.

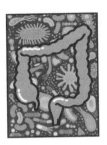

Financial Disclosures

Dr. Chathur Acharya has no financial or proprietary interest in the materials presented herein.

Dr. Jessica R. Allegretti is on the scientific advisory board for Finch Therapeutics and Iterative Scopes; is a consultant for Artugen, Pfizer, Takeda, Janssen, Servatus, and Pandion; and received Grant Support from Merck.

Dr. Olga C. Aroniadis has no financial or proprietary interest in the materials presented herein.

Dr. Jasmohan S. Bajaj has no financial or proprietary interest in the materials presented herein.

Dr. Thomas J. Borody has a pecuniary interest in the Centre for Digestive Diseases, where fecal microbiota transplantation is a treatment option for patients, and he has filed patents in this field.

Dr. Lawrence J. Brandt has no financial or proprietary interest in the materials presented herein.

Dr. Shrish Budree is an employee/shareholder of Finch Therapeutics.

Dr. Jennifer D. Claytor has no financial or proprietary interest in the materials presented herein.

Dr. Suzanne Devkota has no financial or proprietary interest in the materials presented herein.

Dr. Najwa El-Nachef has no financial or proprietary interest in the materials presented herein.

Dr. Paul Feuerstadt is on the speakers bureau at Merck and Co. and a consultant for Ferring Pharmaceuticals and Roche Diagnostics.

Dr. Monika Fischer is a DSMB monitoring board member for Rebiotix and OpenBiome.

Dr. Rohma Ghani has no financial or proprietary interest in the materials presented herein.

Dr. Ari M. Grinspan has no financial or proprietary interest in the materials presented herein.

Dr. Lauren Tal Grinspan has no financial or proprietary interest in the materials presented herein.

Dr. Anoja W. Gunaratne has no financial or proprietary interest in the materials presented herein.

Dr. Zain Kassam is an employee/shareholder of Finch Therapeutics.

Dr. Colleen R. Kelly receives research support from Finch Therapeutics and was a site principal investigator for the PRISM3 clinical trial.

Dr. Alexander Khoruts as research funding from Finch Therapeutics and patents pertaining to preparation and preservation of fecal microbiota for transplantation.

Dr. Joann Kwah has no financial or proprietary interest in the materials presented herein.

Dr. Neena Malik has no financial or proprietary interest in the materials presented herein.

Dr. Paul Moayyedi has no financial or proprietary interest in the materials presented herein.

Dr. Benjamin H. Mullish has received consultancy fees from Finch Therapeutics Group.

Sára Nemes has no financial or proprietary interest in the materials presented herein.

Dr. Majdi Osman is an employee of OpenBiome.

Dr. Pratik Panchal has no financial or proprietary interest in the materials presented herein.

Dr. Abbas Rupawala has no financial or proprietary interest in the materials presented herein.

Dr. Lindsey Russell has no financial or proprietary interest in the materials presented herein.

Dr. Christopher Saddler has no financial or proprietary interest in the materials presented herein.

Dr. Nasia Safdar has no financial or proprietary interest in the materials presented herein.

Dr. Neil Stollman received research grant support from Assembly Bioscience.

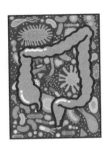

Index